AF904863

ANTIMICROBIAL RESISTANCE - AN OPEN CHALLENGE

Edited by **Maria Cristina Ossiprandi**

Antimicrobial Resistance - An Open Challenge
http://dx.doi.org/10.5772/59829
Edited by Maria Cristina Ossiprandi

Contributors

Maria Cristina Ossiprandi, Laura Zerbini, Marisa De Jesus, Marleen Kock, Ricardo Dos Santos, Marthie Ehlers, Maria Veronica Fernandez-Zenoff, Julian R. Dib, Maria Cristina Estevez, Maria Eugenia Farias, Tracy Schmidt, Kornelia Smalla, Sven Jechalke, Kimberly L Cook

Published by InTech

Janeza Trdine 9, 51000 Rijeka, Croatia

© The Editor(s) and the Author(s) 2015

The moral rights of the editor(s) and the author(s) have been asserted.
All rights to the book as a whole are reserved by InTech. The book as a whole (compilation) cannot be reproduced, distributed or used for commercial or non-commercial purposes without InTech's written permission. Enquiries concerning the use of the book should be directed to InTech's rights and permissions department (permissions@intechopen.com).
Violations are liable to prosecution under the governing Copyright Law.

Individual chapters of this publication are distributed under the terms of the Creative Commons Attribution 3.0 Unported License which permits commercial use, distribution and reproduction of the individual chapters, provided the original author(s) and source publication are appropriately acknowledged. More details and guidelines concerning content reuse and adaptation can be found at http://www.intechopen.com/copyright-policy.html.

Notice

Statements and opinions expressed in the chapters are these of the individual contributors and not necessarily those of the editors or publisher. No responsibility is accepted for the accuracy of information contained in the published chapters. The publisher assumes no responsibility for any damage or injury to persons or property arising out of the use of any materials, instructions, methods or ideas contained in the book.

Publishing Process Manager Iva Lipovic

Technical Editor InTech DTP team

Cover InTech Design team

First published November, 2015

Printed in Croatia

Additional hard copies can be obtained from orders@intechopen.com

Antimicrobial Resistance - An Open Challenge, Edited by Maria Cristina Ossiprandi

p. cm.

ISBN 978-953-51-2222-7

We are IntechOpen, the world's leading publisher of Open Access books

Built by scientists, for scientists

3,800+
Open access books available

116,000+
International authors and editors

120M+
Downloads

151
Countries delivered to

Our authors are among the
Top 1%
most cited scientists

12.2%
Contributors from top 500 universities

BOOK CITATION INDEX
CLARIVATE ANALYTICS
INDEXED

WEB OF SCIENCE™

Selection of our books indexed in the Book Citation Index
in Web of Science™ Core Collection (BKCI)

Interested in publishing with us?
Contact book.department@intechopen.com

Numbers displayed above are based on latest data collected.
For more information visit www.intechopen.com

For EU product safety concerns:
IN TECH d.o.o., Prolaz Marije Krucifikse Kozulić 3, 51000 Rijeka, Croatia,
info@intechopen.com or visit our website at intechopen.com.

Meet the editor

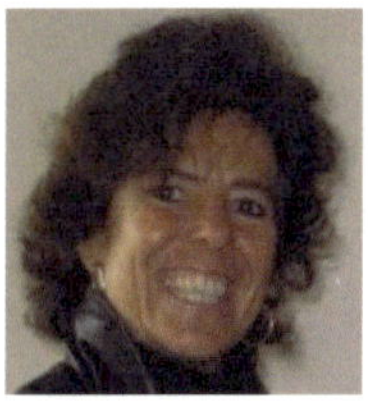

Maria Cristina Ossiprandi graduated in Veterinary Medicine and is Associate Professor (Microbiology and Immunology) in the Department of Veterinary Medical Science, University of Parma, Italy, where she is also Director of the School of Graduate Studies in Animal Health, Breeding and Livestock Production. Until 2010, she was a referee for CINECA and for several scientific journals in the field of microbiology. She is Secretary of AIVEMP (Association involved in Public Medicine in Veterinary).

In November 2013, she was appointed Pro-Rector in Didactic Activities, and in June 2014, she became a representative scientist for an Emilia Romagna (regional) project called Sybilla (predictive microbiology).

In June 2015, she was appointed expert of ANVUR ratings (Disciplinary Expert for the evaluation of degree programs).

She has published a total of 82 papers concerning the epidemiologic studies of potentially zoonotic bacteria in different animal species.

Contents

Preface

The development of antimicrobial resistance in bacteria is universally recognized as a serious threat to public health that goes beyond geographical boundaries and socioeconomic situations. It is a problem that requires a multi-sectorial and global response due to its strong health implications in both human and veterinary medicine.

The reports proposed by the most prestigious and accredited researchers estimate that antimicrobial-resistant infections result in at least 25,000 deaths in 29 European countries and 23,000 deaths in the United States every year.

Furthermore, health costs, due to antibiotic resistance in Europe as well as in the United States, amount to billions of euros that could well be avoided by reducing, contextually, loss in productivity.

The World Health Organization (WHO), together with several governments and other partners, has developed a comprehensive action plan to fight against antimicrobial resistance. This is an essential step involving, on the one hand, the development of national plans in countries that have not yet adopted one and, on the other, the development and strengthening of existing plans. This strategic program must necessarily be supported by constant monitoring fundamental in controlling antibiotic resistance.

This publication responds precisely to this logic by providing a tool that takes into account different bacteria (such as *Staphylococcus aureus* , *Klebsiella* , and *Enterococcus*) that have shown resistance above all to different health environments and epidemiological situations.

The plurality of situations considered (human and veterinary medicine/man and animal), various environments and different substrates offer a case study that is easily viable from a clinical point of view (without forgetting the possible strains resistant between species). WHO has updated its fact sheet concerning the phenomenon of antimicrobial resistance, which clearly points out that there are high rates of antibiotic-resistant microorganisms responsible for common infections (such as urinary tract infections, pneumonia, and bloodstream infections) in regions all over the world.

The winning strategy is most certainly surveillance associated with a proper health education that can be expressed in a "necessary" culture, namely, in virtuous behavior on the part of both the human medical and veterinary worlds: justified use (antibiogram) in clinical cases for which it is essential to resort to antibiotics and appropriate timing of their use (information provided by each pharmaceutical garrison).

It is only thanks to public awareness and continuous monitoring (early detection of any occurrence of resistance and increases in resistance levels) that the phenomenon will be, if not eradicated, at least contained.

Maria Cristina Ossiprandi
Department of Veterinary Medical Science,
Unit of Infectious Diseases and Microbiology,
Parma University, Parma, Italy

Section 1

Antimicrobial Resistance: Impact on Environment and Control

Chapter 1

Water and Flamingo Feces Bacterial Communities from High-Altitude Andean Lakes under Selective Antibiotic Pressure Studied by PCR-DGGE Analyses

María V. Fernández-Zenoff, Julián R. Dib, Anna Neumann,
María C. Estévez and María E. Farías

Additional information is available at the end of the chapter

http://dx.doi.org/10.5772/61967

Abstract

High-altitude Andean lakes are exposed to extreme environmental factors like high salinity, ultraviolet radiation, heavy metals, among others. As it was previously shown, these lakes are not only the habitat of a high diversity of bacteria with multiple resistances; they also support an enormous population of flamingos, which migrate among these wetlands, and they could play a role as disseminators and/or reservoirs of pathogenic bacteria.

The aim of this work was to analyze, by Denaturant Gradient Gel Electrophoresis, the bacterial population under selective antibiotic pressure from bacterioplankton and flamingo feces from three lakes, placed between altitudes 4,200 and 4,560 m. Almost all bands were present in antibiotic-enriched cultures. Several bands identified in water were found in feces as well, presenting mainly correspondence with *Gamma-proteobacteria*. Few bands were exclusively identified in water, and those presenting correspondence with *Alfa-proteobacteria* and Actinobacteria were only identified in Laguna Azul.

This study established that flamingos' enteric biota is in close interaction with lake water and demonstrated that bacteria with the ability to grow in antibiotics are abundant and diverse in the microbiota of Andean lakes. Additionally, flamingos could be considered as vectors of pathogenic organisms, since *Stenotrophomonas* seem to be the widest spread bacteria in the studied lakes.

Keywords: Andean Lakes, Antibiotics, DGGE, Flamingos, Feces, Resistance

1. Introduction

High-Altitude Andean Lakes (HAAL) are a system of shallow oligotrophic lakes originated in the tertiary age distributed across the *Puna,* the highest plateau of the South American Andes

INTECH
open science | open minds

© 2015 The Author(s). Licensee InTech. This chapter is distributed under the terms of the Creative Commons Attribution License (http://creativecommons.org/licenses/by/3.0), which permits unrestricted use, distribution, and reproduction in any medium, provided the original work is properly cited.

that includes Peru, Bolivia, Chile, and Argentina. These lakes are scattered throughout the region at altitudes varying from 3,600 to 6,000 m above sea level. As it was described in previous works done by our group, HAAL are almost unexplored environments, most of them with no access roads; they are distant from each other (more than 500–700 km) and the unique connection among them would be flamingo migration. Furthermore, they are exposed to extreme conditions, such as high salinity, UV radiation, oligotrophy with low phosphor availability, daily temperature changes (-15ºC to 20ºC), and heavy metal content [1-6]. HAAL are home to large flocks of aquatic birds, mainly flamingos. Three of the six extant flamingo species coexist in HAAL: the James's Flamingo (*Phoenicopterus jamesi*), the Chilean Flamingo (*Phoenicopterus chilensis*), and the Andean Flamingo (*Phoenicopterus andinus*). James's flamingos are distributed primarily in the Andean wetlands, during the breeding season, and dispersed through the lowland wetlands in Argentina in winter, during the nonbreeding season, when some of the high-Andes lakes freeze [7-9]. The Chilean flamingo inhabits most of the Pampean lowland wetlands throughout the year. Both flamingo species have specialized beaks that allow them to filter and feed on many planktonic and benthic organisms [10]. Migratory birds are known to play a role as long-distance vectors for many microorganisms, and antimicrobial drug resistance has also been described in bacteria isolated from wild birds [11-15]. In previous publications carried out in our laboratory we demonstrated that bacteria isolated from water and flamingo feces from HAAL were resistant to at least three or more antibiotics (ATBs) [2, 3]. However, the response of the whole community to antibiotic pressure using molecular methods has never been studied.

In this chapter, we compare bacterial diversity using Denaturant Gradient Gel Electrophoresis (DGGE) under antibiotic pressure conditions in water and flamingo feces from three HAAL: Laguna Aparejos, Laguna Negra, and Laguna Azul.

2. Materials and methods

2.1. Description of environments and sampling

Aparejos, Negra, and Azul lakes are located in the Andes Mountains in the northwest of Argentina; their physic and chemical characteristics are described by Dib et al. [3]. They are a group of lakes and salar pads called Salar de la Laguna Verde in the Andean region of Catamarca province, Argentina (27º 34′ S; 68º 32′ W). Some of the highest mountains of the Andean system are located in this area: Ojos del Salado (6,885 m) and Nevado Pissis (6,779 m). The water temperature was 5ºC at the sampling time (1 pm local hour) and the maximal UV-B irradiance reached 3.3 Wm^{-2} for 312 nm (half band with 300–325 nm).

Two types of samples were considered: water and flamingo feces. Surface water samples were collected during summer 2009 (near the beginning of austral spring) in 10 L sterile polyethylene bottles. Water samples were stored at 4ºC until further processing in the laboratory (within 24 h after collection), which is located 600 km away from the sampling site. Flamingo feces were taken near the lake and conserved in sterile bags at 4ºC until processing. Once in a sterile environment in the lab, core feces samples were extracted for cultivation.

2.2. Antibiotics-resistant bacteria-enrichment cultures

To determine bacterial diversity under selective pressure, water samples from Laguna Aparejos, Laguna Negra, Laguna Azul, and four flamingo feces samples from each lake were analyzed. Samples were inoculated in 20 mL of R2A medium (yeast extract 0.5 g L^{-1}, peptone 0.5 g L^{-1}, casamino acids 0.5 g L^{-1}, glucose 0.5 g L^{-1}, soluble starch 0.5 g L^{-1}, sodium pyruvate 0.3 g L^{-1}, K_2HPO_4 0.3 g L^{-1}, $MgSO_4{\times}7H_2O$ 0.05 g L^{-1}; pH 7.2), with different ATBs. Control cultures without ATBs were also performed. Five ATBs were used: ampicillin (Amp), 100 μg mL^{-1}; chloramphenicol (Cm), 170 μg mL^{-1}; colistin (Col), 20 μg mL^{-1}; erythromycin (Ery), 50 μg mL^{-1}; and tetracycline (Tet) 50 μg mL^{-1}. After five days of incubation at 30ºC and 150 rpm, the cells were pelleted by centrifugation and total DNA was extracted from the ATB enriched cultures. Afterward, DGGE profiles of total community cultured without or with different ATBs were determined.

2.3. PCR amplification DGGE and sequencing

DNA extraction from total community cultures was performed using a CTAB method [16]. The variable V3 region of 16S rRNA gene was amplified by PCR [17]. The nucleotide sequences of the primers are as follows: primer 1 F341: 5′-CGC CCG CCG CGC CCC GCG CCC GTC CCG CCG CCC CCG CCC GCC TAC GGG AGG CAG CAG-3′, primer 2 R518: 5′-CGT ATT ACC GCG GCT GCT GG-3′, primer 3 F357: 5′-TTA CTG ATA GAA TGT GGA GC-3′[18].

PCR amplification was performed with a Biometra Termocycler as follows: 100 ηg of purified genomic DNA, 20 pmol of each primers (Genbiotech), 200 μmol of each deoxyribonucleoside triphosphate, 10 μL of 10× PCR buffer ($MgCl_2$) and 0.25 U of Go Taq polymerase (Promega) were added to a 0.2 mL volume microtube, which was filled up to a volume of 25 μL with sterile Milli-Q-water. PCR was performed using the following conditions: initial denaturing step of 15 min at 95°C, followed by 30 cycles of 95°C for 1 min, 65°C for 1 min, and 72°C for 1 min 30 s. A touchdown program was performed in order to down one grade at each cycle, until 55ºC. At this last temperature, 15 additional cycles were programmed, with a final extension at 72°C for 5 min. DGGE was performed with the Bio-Rad Protean II system, essentially as described previously [19]. PCR products were applied directly onto 8% (wt/vol) polyacrylamide gels in 1X TAE buffer (40 mM Tris base, 20 mM sodium acetate, 1 mM EDTA) and a linear gradient consisting of the denaturants urea and formamide; the concentration of the denaturants increased from 40% at the top of the gel to 60% at the bottom. Electrophoresis was performed at a constant voltage of 120 V and a temperature of 60ºC during 5 h. After electrophoresis, the gel was stained for 10 min with SYBR® Gold (Molecular Probes, Eugene, OR), rinsed with TAE buffer, and visualized with a Bio-Rad UV Gel Doc 2000 transilluminator. Distinguishable bands were excised from the gel; the eluted DNA was reamplified using the primers 2 and 3, and PCR products were sequenced.

2.4. Nucleotide sequence accession numbers and data analysis

Fifty-nine selected 16S rRNA sequences from DGGE bands in this paper have been deposited in GenBank database under the following accession numbers: AM712052–66, AM711573–79, AM711878–90, and AM889064–87.

The similarity in DGGE bands in each lake was assessed by Cluster Analysis using the Jaccard's index, applying the UPGMA (unweight pair-group method using averages) algorithm with software MVSP 3.2.

3. Results

3.1. Diversity of ATB-resistant bacteria in water and feces

The affiliation of the prominent reamplified bands from DGGE gels from major bacterial community members obtained from ATB enrichment cultures, from water and feces, in all studied lakes is shown in Table 1. 16S rRNA gene sequence comparisons revealed that most of the water and feces DGGE bands were represented mainly by *Proteobacteria,* particularly, *Gamma-proteobacteria,* which is grouped among typical planktonic bacteria, but also *Alpha-proteobacteria* and *Beta-proteobacteria. Gamma-proteobacteria* group is represented by *Pseudomonadales, Aeromonadales,* and *Xanthomonadales* members in Aparejos, Negra, and Azul lakes, in both water and feces samples.

Band sequences related to *Beta-proteobacteria,* belonged mainly to *Burkholderiales* (*Comamonas* sp., *Curvibacter* sp., and *Duganella* sp.) members, were recovered from Aparejos and Azul samples. Bands sequences related to *Alpha-proteobacteria* group were only recovered from Azul samples. The presence of Firmicutes was indicated by several DGGE bands in the three studied lakes, most of them grouped among *Bacillales, Clostridiales,* and *Lactobacillales* members.

In Laguna Aparejos, two bands sequences (A15 and A18) were exclusively recovered from water and they presented similarities with members of the genera *Enterobacter* and *Commamonas*.

The sequence related to *Stenotrophomonas* was the most widespread among all lakes, in both water and bird feces samples, since sixteen band sequences were matched to this genus.

Phylogenetic Group	DGGE Bands Closest Identified Relative (Accession Number)	% Similarity	Source	ATBs Resistances
Laguna Aparejos				
Beta-proteobacteria				
A16	*Duganella* sp. (AM711889)	90	F, W	Col
A18	*Comamonas* sp. (AM711890)	98	W	Amp
Gamma-proteobacteria				
A1	*Pantoea* sp. (AM711573)	100	W, F	Amp, Col, Ery Cm, Tet
A2; A3; A4A; A16a, A5A	*Stenotrophomonas* sp. (AM711575; AM711576; AM711577; AM711888; AM711577)	96-100	W, F	Amp, Ery, Cm, Tet
A9; A10; A14; A8A	*Pseudomonas* sp. (AM711878;AM711879; AM711886; AM711579)	98-100	W, F	Amp, Ery, Col, Tet
A2A	*Pseudomonas* sp. (AM711574)	98	F	Amp
A13	*Klebsiella* sp. (AM711884)	95	W, F	Amp, Ery

Phylogenetic Group	DGGE Bands Closest Identified Relative (Accession Number)	% Similarity	Source	ATBs Resistances
A15	*Enterobacter* sp. (AM711887)	98	W	Amp, Col, Tet
A13a	*Acinetobacter* sp. (AM711883)	98	F	Amp, Ery, Cm, Tet
Firmicutes				
A11a	*Carnobacterium* sp. (AM711880)	96	F	
A11	*Enterococcus* sp. (AM711881)	98	F	Col
A14a	*Clostridium* sp. (AM711885)	99	F	
A12a	*Bacillus* sp. (AM711882)	97	F	
Laguna Negra				
Gamma-proteobacteria				
N1	*Aeromonas* sp. (AM712052)	97	W, F	Amp, Col
N2	*Enterobacter* sp. (AM712053)	99	W, F	Amp, Col
N8; N5	*Escherichia* sp. (AM712056; AM712054)	96-99	F	Amp
N10; N11; N11a; N12	*Rahnella* sp. (AM712058; AM712060; AM712059; AM712061)	99	W, F	Amp, Col
N13; N14	*Aeromonas* sp. (AM712062; AM712063)	95-99	W, F	Amp, Col, Tet
N16; N19	*Stenotrophomonas* sp. (AM712065; AM712066)	99-100	W	Col, Ery, Tet
Firmicutes				
N6	*Clostridium* sp. (AM712055)	99	F	Amp
N9; N15	*Bacillus* sp. (AM712057; AM712064)	99-100	F	Amp, Col
Laguna Azul				
Alpha-proteobacteria				
Az1; Az14	*Sphingomonas* sp. (AM889064; AM889077)	92-95	W	Amp, Col, Tet
Beta-proteobacteria				
Az11	*Curvibacter* sp. (AM889074)	98	F	Cm, Tet
Az9	*Delftia* sp.(AM889072)	99	F	Col
Az16; Az18	*Variovorax* sp. (AM889079; AM889081)	96	F	Col, Tet
Gamma-proteobacteria				
Az4	*Pseudomonas* sp.(AM889067)	83	W	Col
Az19; Az20; Az2;	*Pseudomonas* sp. (AM889082; AM889083; AM889065;	96-99	W, F	Amp
Az6; Az15; Az10; Az21; Az8; Az25; Az23; Az7; Az17	*Stenotrophomonas* sp.(AM889069; AM889078; AM889073; AM889084; AM889071; AM889087; AM889085; AM889070; AM889080)	96-99	F	Amp, Ery, Tet
Firmicutes				
Az24	*Bacillus* sp.(AM889086)	96	F	Ery
Az13; Az12; Az3	*Bacillus* sp.(AM889076; AM889075; AM889066)	98-100	W, F	Ery, Amp, Col
Actinobacteria				
Az5	*Arthrobacter* sp. (AM889068)	96	F	

Table 1. Phylogenetic affiliation of sequences obtained from DGGE bands from water (W) and feces (F).

3.2. Antibiotics resistances

The microbial diversity by DGGE in water and feces after cultivation under antimicrobial pressure could be explained by the presence of ATB-resistant traits or the acquisition of resistant traits by horizontal gene transfer events during cultivation.

In Laguna Aparejos, there was a band sequence detected in the five enrichment cultures conditions. It was the case of a band sequence related to *Pantoea* sp. This band sequence was found in water as well as feces samples in all ATB tested. Another example of an extensive ATB resistance to tested ATB was those of band sequences (A13a) matched with *Acinetobacter* sp.

In Laguna Negra, most of the DGGE-detected bands were found in Col- and Amp-enriched cultures. Two band sequences (N13, N14) matched with *Aeromonas* sp. were detected in enrichment cultures with Amp, Col, and Tet. Two band sequences related to *Stenotrophomonas* (N16, N19) were the only ones that depicted resistance to Ery in this lake. In Laguna Azul, there were bands detected in all of the ATB enrichment culture tested. However, there was one band sequence that matched with *Arthrobacter* sp. (Az5) that was not visible in any ATB-enriched culture but only in control culture for feces.

DGGE band sequences matched with *Stenotrophomonas* were present in all studied lakes; however, their "ATB resistance profile" was different among them. While in Aparejos it was recovered from Amp, Ery, Cm, and Tet enrichment culture, in Negra, resistances included Col, Ery and Tet, while in Azul Lake, the ATB profile included Amp, Ery, and Tet.

3.3. DGGE analyses

Figure 1 shows the dendrogram resulting from the Cluster Analysis performed among samples taking into account the presence or absence of individual bands obtained by DGGE profiles of Laguna Aparejos. The analysis evidenced that water and flamingo feces without any antimicrobial pressure clustered together conforming a subgroup.

In Laguna Negra, cluster analysis indicates that water, feces, and feces with Amp clustered within the same subgroup (Figure 2).

In Laguna Azul, two clear groups can be observed, one for feces samples and the other for water samples (Figure 3).

4. Discussion

It was proposed that landscape ecology, which links the biotic and abiotic factors of an ecosystem, might help to untangle the complexity of antibiotic resistance and improve the interpretation of ecological studies [20]. Continuing that idea, we have previously demonstrated that water in high-irradiated pristine environments was a source for isolating bacteria able to grow in the presence of antibiotics, and that the bacteria were also present in flamingos' enteric biota, probably taken from the water where they feed [3]. In addition, we have found

http://dx.doi.org/10.5772/61967

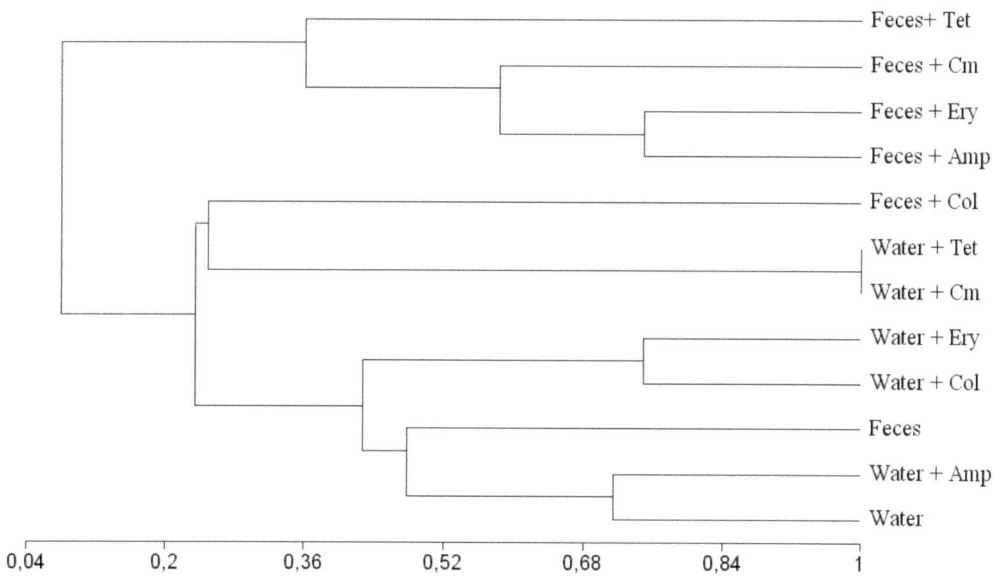

Figure 1. Clustering using band-based Jaccard coefficient for Laguna Aparejos samples.

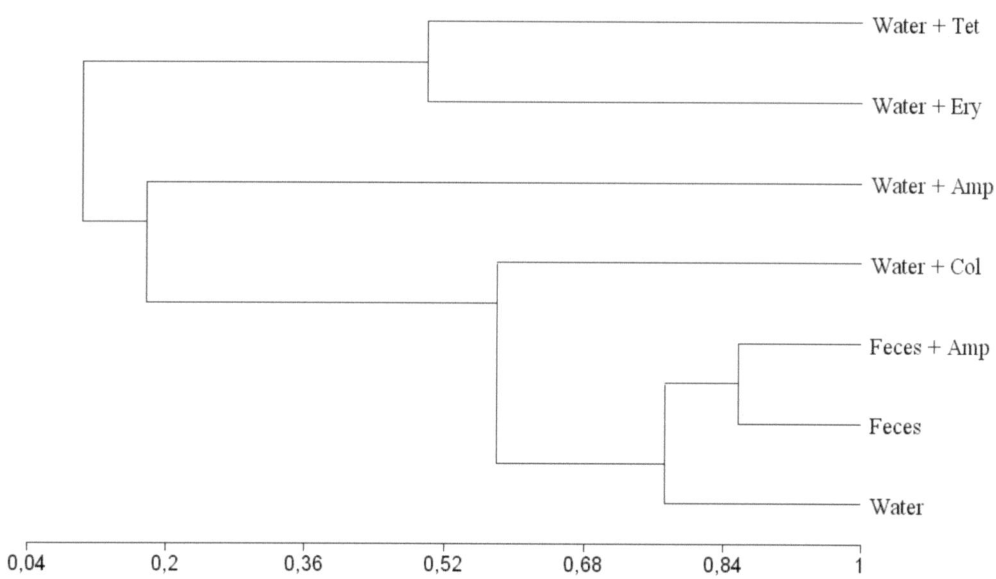

Figure 2. UPGMA dendrogram resulting from the Cluster Analysis performed among samples from Laguna Negra.

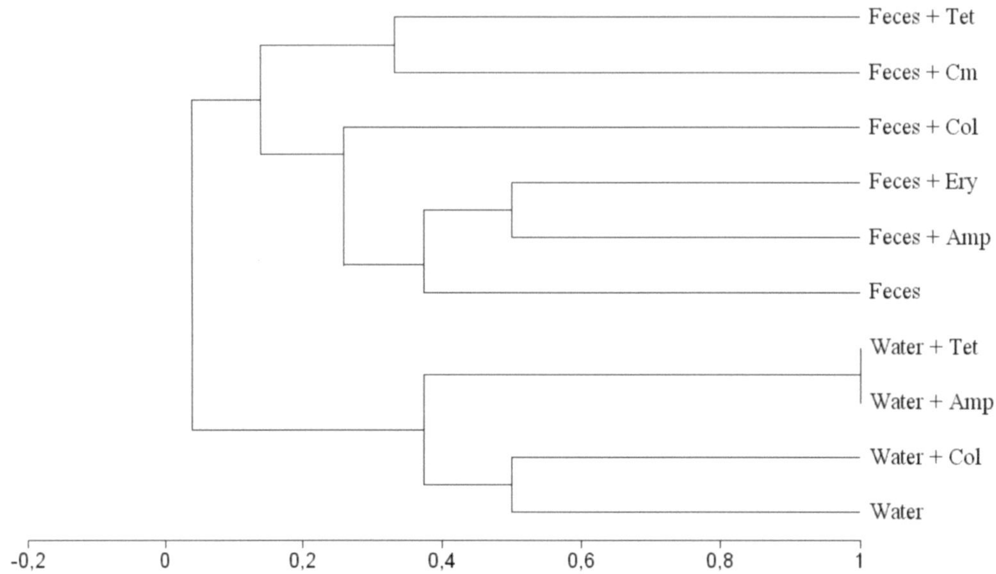

Figure 3. Dendrogram based in Jaccard coefficient showing the similarity coefficient of bacterial community from enrichment ATBs cultures from water and flamingo feces.

that several isolated bacteria present giant extra chromosomal linear elements, the so-called linear plasmids [21-23]. We found that the presence of linear plasmids might be related to the antibiotics-resistant dispersion. In this work, we attempt to study the total bacterial community under different selective pressures and the connection between the microbiota associated to lake water and flamingo feces.

4.1. Antibiotic-resistant bacteria is an spread phenomenon in high-altitude lakes

We showed that the ability to grow in ATB or the rapid spread of this ability was abundant, diverse, and widely distributed in the water and feces of the studied high-altitude environments. As it was postulated by our group in previous publications [2, 3], UV radiation would be in connection with ATB resistances since under extreme UV stress, bacteria are known to increase mutational events, through a resistance mechanism named error-prone repair [24]. In many cases, spontaneous resistance to ATB is known to emerge under such mutagenic conditions, as consequence of mutagenesis modified potential target genes. In addition, a possible connection of oxidative stress resistances and an association with ATB resistances were also established [25]. As it was largely established that UV radiation produces high oxidative stress, thus a high-irradiated environment is expected to select oxidative stress-resistant bacteria, and this could also be in connection with ATB resistances found in more irradiated environments.

One the other hand, exposure of wild birds to human-generated wastewater presents a pathway for transfer of bacteria and the antibiotic resistance genes that they carry [26]. Water bodies of Pampean Lakes are threatened by many anthropic activities, resulting from land use, agriculture, and livestock, with the subsequent deposition of a significant amount of organic wastes, fertilizers, and pesticides [27-30]. Therefore, flamingos exposed to such sources could be colonized by microorganisms that are not typical of their natural habitats and are involved in the dissemination of multidrug-resistant bacteria since migration of flamingos, among lakes from Andean lakes in summer to Pampean lakes in winter, is an established phenomenon [31]. Our next challenge is subject to deeper studies the flamingo's role as disseminators and/or reservoir of multidrug-resistant bacteria.

4.2. Microbiota in water and birds feces

Mostly, band sequences identified in water samples were also found in feces. Thus we observed a connection between the bacterial community's inhabitant flamingos intestinal and those of the water lake, where these birds obtain their food: community structure harboring similar ATB resistances were similar in both water and feces samples, sampled from the same lake. Special attention should be given to *Stenotrophomonas,* since it seems to be the widest spread bacterium. It was detected in DGGE bands of water and feces of Aparejos, Negra, and Azul lakes and isolated from water and feces of Negra and Azul lakes and, in all the cases, it was the most resistant to multiple ATB [2]. This bacterium has been increasingly recognized as an important cause of nosocomial infection. Infection occurs principally, but not exclusively, in debilitated and immunosuppressed individuals. The management of *S. maltophilia* infections is often problematic because this pathogen is frequently inherently resistant to multiple antibiotics [32, 33].

A band corresponding to *Acinetobacter* sp. was also detected in Laguna Aparejos. In previous reports we showed *Acinetobacter* strains that offer high ATB and UV resistance [1, 2, 16, 34, 35] and also other related strains from water and feces of Negra, Azul, and Vilama with multiple ATB resistances [5].

As it was determined by our preview reports [2, 3], we confirm the idea that pathogenic organism resistant to multi-antibiotics are not a phenomena restricted to spoiled environments and that pristine environments could be considered as important reservoirs of bacteria like *Klebsiella pneumoniae, Staphylococcus* sp., *Aeromonas* sp., *S. maltophilia,* and a wide group of enteric bacteria resistant to multiple ATB. Birds with wide migration itineraries could indeed spread these bacteria. Thus, from an epidemiological point of view, pristine UV-irradiated environments should receive more attention as reservoirs of potential human pathogens as well as ATB resistances.

Nomenclatures

HAAL – High Altitude Andean Lakes; ATBs – Antibiotics; DGGE – Denaturant Gradient Gel Electrophoresis

Acknowledgements

This work was supported by PIE CONICET 6268-6096, Fundación Antorchas Nº 14248-133, PICT-Agencia Nacional de Promoción Científica y Tecnológica Nº14498. María Verónica Fernández-Zenoff is recipient of a CONICET fellowship. Anna Neumann received financial support from DAAD.

Author details

María V. Fernández-Zenoff[1,3*], Julián R. Dib[1,3], Anna Neumann[2], María C. Estévez[1] and María E. Farías[1]

*Address all correspondence to: verozenoff@hotmail.com

1 Planta Piloto de Procesos Industriales Microbiológicos (PROIMI -CONICET), Tucumán, Argentina

2 Technische Universität Berlin, Berlin, Germany

3 Instituto de Microbiología, Facultad de Bioquímica, Química y Farmacia, Universidad Nacional de Tucumán, Tucumán, Argentina

References

[1] Zenoff VF, Heredia J, Ferrero MA, Siñeriz F, Farías ME. Diverse UV-B resistance of culturable bacterial community from high-altitude wetland water. *Curr Microbiol.* 2006;52: 359-362. DOI: 10.1007/s00284-005-0241-5

[2] Dib J, Motok J, Fernandez Zenoff V, Ordoñez O, Farías ME. Occurrence of resistance to antibiotics, UV-B and arsenic in bacteria isolated from extreme environments in high altitude (above 4,400 m) Andean lakes. *Curr Microbiol.* 2008;56(5):510-517. DOI: 10.1007/s00284-008-9103-2

[3] Dib JR, Weiss A, Neumann A, Ordoñez O, Estévez MC, Farías ME. Isolation of bacteria from remote high altitude Andean lakes able to grow in the presence of antibiotics. *Recent Patents Anti-Infect Drug Discov.* 2009;4(1): 66-76. DOI: 10.2174/157489109787236300

[4] Farias ME, Fernández-Zenoff MV, Flores MR, Ordoñez OF, Estevez MC. Impact of solar radiation on bacterioplankton in Laguna Vilama, a hypersaline Andean saline lake (4,650 m). *J Geophysic Res.* 2009;114:G00D04. DOI:10.1029/2008JG000784

[5] Ordoñez OF, Flores MR, Dib JR, Paz A, Farías ME. Extremophile culture collection from Andean lakes: extreme pristine environments that host a wide diversity of microorganisms with tolerance to UV radiation. *Microb Ecol.*2009; 58:461-473. DOI: 10.1007/s00248-009-9527-7

[6] AlbarracínVH, Dib JR, Ordoñez OF, Farías ME. A harsh life to indigenous *proteobacteria* at the Andean mountains: microbial diversity and resistance mechanisms towards extreme conditions. In: Sezenna ML editor. *Proteobacteria: Phylogeny, Metabolic Diversity and Ecological Effects*. Nova Science Publishers, Inc.; 2011. p. 91-131.

[7] Caziani SM, Rocha Olivio O, Rodriguez Ramirez E, Romano M, Derlindati EJ, Talamo A, Ricalde D, Quiroga C, Contreras JP, Valqui M, Sosa H. Mint: Seasonal distribution, abundance, and nesting of Puna, Andean, and Chilean Flamingos. *The Condor*. 2007;109(2):276-287. DOI: http://dx.doi.org/10.1650/0010-5422(2007)109[276:SDAANO]2.0.CO;2

[8] Romano M, Barberis IMM, Derlindati EJ, Pagano F, Marconi P, Arengo F. Variation in abundance of Andean and Chilean Flamingos wintering in lowland wetlands of central Argentina in two contrasting years. *Flamingo*. 2009;17: 11-16.

[9] Cruz NN, Barisón C, Romano M, Arengo F, Derlindati EJ, Barberis I. A new record of James's Flamingo (*Phoenicoparrus jamesi*) from Laguna Melincué, a lowland wetland in east-central Argentina. *Wilson J Ornithol.* 2013;125(1):217-221. DOI: http://dx.doi.org/10.1676/12-111.1

[10] Hurlbert SH. Limnological studies of flamingo diets and distributions. *Natl Geographic Res*. 1982;14:351-356.

[11] Benskin CMcWH, Wilson K, Jones K, Hartley IR. Bacterial pathogens in wild birds: a review of the frequency and effects of infection. *Biologic Rev.* 2009;84:349-373. DOI: 10.1111/j.1469-185X.2008.00076.x

[12] Cole D, Drum DJV, Stallknecht DE, White DG, Lee MD, Ayers S, Sobsey M, Maurer JJ. Free-living Canada geese and antimicrobial resistance. *Emerging Infect Dis.* 2005;11:935-938. DOI: 10.3201/eid1106.040717

[13] Middleton JH, Ambrose A. Enumeration and antibiotic resistance patterns of fecal indicator organisms isolated from migratory Canada Geese (*Branta canadensis*). *J Wildlife Dis.* 2005;41:334-341. DOI: http://www.bioone.org/doi/full/10.7589/0090-3558-41.2.334Miglioranza KS, Moreno JEAD, Moreno VJ. Trends in soil science: Organochlorine pesticides in Argentinean soils. *J Soils Sediments*. 2003;3(4): 264-265. DOI: 10.1007/BF02988686

[14] Sjölund M, Bonnedahl J, Hernandez J, Bengtsson S, Cederbrant G, Pinhassi J, Kahlmeter G, Olsen B. Dissemination of multidrug-resistant bacteria into the Arctic. *Emerging Infect Dis*. 2008;14: 70-72. DOI: 10.3201/eid1401.070704

[15] Hatha AAM, Divya PS, Saramma, AV, Rahiman M, Krishnan KP. Migratory bird, *Branta leucopis* (Barnacle goose), a potential carrier of diverse *Escherichia coli* serotypes into pristine Arctic environment. *Curr Sci.* 2013;104(8):1078.

[16] Fernández Zenoff V, Siñeriz F, Farias ME. Diverse responses to UV-B radiation and repair mechanisms of bacteria isolated from high-altitude aquatic environments. *Appl Environ Microbiol.* 2006;72(12): 7857-7863. DOI: 10.1128/AEM.01333-06

[17] Saiki RK, Scharf SJ, Faloona F, Mullis KB, Horn GT, Erlich HA, Arnheim N. Enzymatic amplification of beta-globin genomic sequences and restriction site analysis for diagnosis of sickle cell anemia. *Science.* 1985,230: 1350-1354. DOI: 10.1126/science.2999980

[18] Medlin L, Elwood HJ, Stickel S, Sogin ML. The characterization of enzymatically amplified eukaryotic 16S-like rRNA coding regions. *Gene.* 1998;71:491-499. DOI: 10.1016/0378-1119(88)90066-2

[19] Fischer SG, Lerman LS. DNA fragments differing by single basepair substitutions are separated in denaturing gradient gels: correspondence with melting theory. *Proc Natl Acad Sci.* 1983;80:1579-1583.

[20] Singer RS, Ward MP, Maldonado G. Can landscape ecology untangle the complexity of antibiotic resistance? *Natur Rev Microbiol.* 2006;4: 943-952. DOI: 10.1038/nrmicro1553

[21] Dib JR, Liebl W, Wagenknecht M, Farías ME, Meinhardt F. Extrachromosomal genetic elements in *Micrococcus*. *Appl Microbiol Biotechnol.* 2013;97(1):63-75. DOI: 10.1007/s00253-012-4539-5

[22] Dib JR, Schuldes J, Thürmer A, Farias ME, Daniel R, Meinhardt F. Complete genome sequence of pAP13, a large linear plasmid of a *Brevibacterium* strain isolated from a saline lake at 4,200 meters above sea level in Argentina. *Genome Announce.* 2013;1(6), e00878-13. DOI:10.1128/genomeA.00878-13.

[23] Dib JR, Schuldes J, Thürmer A, Farias ME, Daniel R, Meinhardt F. First complete sequence of a giant linear plasmid from a *Micrococcus* strain isolated from an extremely high-altitude lake. *Genome Announce.* 2013;1(6):e00885-13. DOI:10.1128/genomeA.00885-13.

[24] Smith BT, Walker GC. Mutagenesis and more: umuDC and the *Escherichia coli* SOS response. *Genetics.* 1998;148: 1599-1610.

[25] Ariza RR, Li Z, Ringstad N, Demple B. Activation of multiple antibiotic resistance and binding of stress-inducible promoters by *Escherichia coli* Rob protein. *J Bacteriol.* 1995;177(7):1655-1661.

[26] Pellegrini C, Mercuri PS, Celenza G, Galleni M, Segatore B, Sacchetti E, Volpe R, Amicosante G, Perilli M. Identification of bla(IMP-22) in *Pseudomonas* spp. in urban wastewater andnosocomial environments: biochemical characterization of a new

IMP metalloenzyme variant and its genetic location. *J Antimicrob Chemother*. 2009;63:901-908. DOI: 10.1093/jac/dkp061

[27] Romano M, Barberis I, Pagano F, Maidagan J. Seasonal and interannual variation in waterbird abundance and species composition in the Melincué saline lake, Argentina. *Eur J Wildlife Res*. 2005;51(1): 1-13. DOI: 10.1007/s10344-005-0078-z

[28] Pengue, W. 2005. Agricultura industrial y agricultura familiar en el Mercosur: el pez grande se come al chico... siempre? *Le Monde Diplomatique, Edición Cono Sur*. 2005;71: 7–9.

[29] Peruzzo PJ, Porta AAA, Ronco AE. Levels of glyphosate in surface waters, sediments and soils associated with direct sowing soybean cultivation in north pampasic region of Argentina. *Environ Poll*. 2008;156(1): 61-66. DOI: 10.1016/j.envpol.2008.01.015

[30] Coconier E. Reporte final aves acuáticas en la Argentina. In: Blanco DE, editor. *La Conservación de las Aves Acuáticas para las Américas* (*Waterbird Conservation for the Americas*). Wetlands Int. Buenos Aires, Argentina. 2005. p. 2-137.

[31] Denton M, Kerr KG. Microbiological and clinical aspects of infection associated with *Stenotrophomonas maltophilia*. *Clin Microbiol Rev*.1998;11:57-80.

[32] Mercuri PS, Ishii Y, Ma L, Rossolini GM, Luzzaro F, Amicosante G, Franceschini N, Frere JM, Galleni M. Clonal diversity and metallo-β-lactamase production in clinical isolates of *Stenotrophomonas maltophilia*. *Microb Drug Resist*. 2002;8(3):193-200. DOI: 10.1089/107662902760326904

[33] Di Capua C, Bortolotti A, Farías ME, Cortez N. UV-resistant *Acinetobacter* sp. isolates from Andean wetlands display high catalase activity. *FEMS Microbiol Lett*. 2011;317(2):181-189. DOI: http://dx.doi.org/10.1111/j.1574-6968.2011.02231.x

[34] Albarracín VH, Pathak GP, Douki T, Cadet J, Borsarelli CD, Gärtner W, Farias ME. Extremophilic *Acinetobacter* strains from high-altitude lakes in Argentinean Puna: remarkable UV-B resistance and efficient DNA damage repair. Origin Life Evol Biospheres. 2012;42: 201-221. DOI: 10.1007/s11084-012-9276-3

Chapter 2

Approaches to Assess the Effects and Risks of Veterinary Antibiotics Applied with Manure to Soil

Sven Jechalke, Kimberly L. Cook and Kornelia Smalla

Additional information is available at the end of the chapter

http://dx.doi.org/10.5772/61871

Abstract

In veterinary medicine, large quantities of antibiotic substances are administered each year for therapeutic and prophylactic purposes or to promote growth. As a consequence, the antibiotics and bacteria carrying transferable antibiotic resistance genes are excreted by the animals and reach the environment through run-off, leaching, and/or following manure application to agricultural fields, where they have been found to affect the structure and function of soil bacterial communities. However, we are only beginning to understand the global effects of environmental pollution with antibiotics and resistance determinants and the resulting risks for human health. For regulatory purposes, there is urgent need for criteria and methods that allow reliable and reproducible assessment of risks associated with release of realistic concentrations of antibiotics and resistance determinants into the environment following manure application. In this chapter, we will summarize recent advances, limitations, and research needed to optimize the methods to quantify and evaluate the effects and risks associated with these compounds. Approaches that are discussed focus on antibiotic resistance genes and include classical tools such as cultivation and PCR detection as well as quantitative real-time PCR and next-generation sequencing technologies used in combination with functional screening.

Keywords: Antibiotic resistance, resistome, manure, soil, mobilome

1. Introduction

Antibiotic-resistant pathogens are a growing public health threat challenging the achievements of modern medicine by making available treatment options for common infections ineffective.[1] It is widely accepted that this rise in antibiotic-resistant bacteria is due to the massive and worldwide use, misuse, and abuse of antibiotic agents in humans and animals. Additionally, antibiotics are applied prophylactically to control bacterial diseases of plants,

INTECH
open science | open minds

© 2015 The Author(s). Licensee InTech. This chapter is distributed under the terms of the Creative Commons Attribution License (http://creativecommons.org/licenses/by/3.0), which permits unrestricted use, distribution, and reproduction in any medium, provided the original work is properly cited.

especially fire blight of pear and apple and bacterial spot of peach.[2] Besides clinical and agricultural use, large quantities of antibiotic substances are administered each year in veterinary medicine for therapeutic and prophylactic purposes or in different parts of the world still to promote growth.[3,4] Depending on pharmacokinetics and specific transformation processes in the animals, large proportions of antibiotics and antibiotic-resistant bacteria (often with resistance determinants located on mobile genetic elements) are typically excreted by the animals. Ultimately, these components reach the environment via run-off, leaching, and/or manure application, where they at least transiently affect the structure and function of soil bacterial communities.[5–8]

Recent studies have demonstrated the existence of a shared antibiotic resistome between clinical pathogens and the environmental bacteria.[9–11] Thus, although the observed increase in abundance and transferability of antibiotic resistance genes in manured soil is assumed to be only transient, it is very likely that the pollution of the environment with antibiotics and antibiotic resistance determinants influences the human microbiome and contributes to the rise of antibiotic resistance found in human pathogens.[12,13] Mobile genetic elements such as plasmids are considered to play an important role in the adaptation of bacterial communities facing selective pressure by antibiotics[14,15] and might be an important link between the environmental and human resistome. Co-selection processes by heavy metals such as copper and zinc[16] or by disinfectants such as quaternary ammonium compounds (QACs)[17,18] can further promote the spread and persistence of antibiotic resistance genes on similar genetic platforms. Moreover, the rhizosphere of plants is considered to increase the horizontal transfer of resistance determinants within bacterial communities and to modify the effects of antibiotics applied with manure by root exudates that affect the bacterial cell density, distribution, and metabolic activity (reviewed by Jechalke et al.[5]).

Nevertheless, little is known regarding the global effects of environmental pollution with antibiotics and resistance determinants by manure fertilization and the resulting risks for human health. To extend the time that antibiotics can be effectively used in human and veterinary medicine, agricultural management options are necessary to reduce the environmental release and spread of antibiotics and antibiotic resistance determinants. Policy makers are focusing on agricultural sources of antibiotic resistance as a result of recent reports that emphasize the importance of antibiotic resistance in environmental bacteria (pathogenic and non-pathogenic) as a point source for spread to environmental and human ecosystems.[6,19–24] These findings, coupled with the potential for spread of emergent antibiotic-resistant bacteria from livestock to human populations and the lack of new antibiotics entering the market, have placed pressure on the agricultural community, increasing the urgency for science-based studies that fill gaps in current knowledge about how antibiotic resistance spreads within environmental ecosystems. Furthermore, on a policy level, there is urgent need for criteria and methods that allow reliable and reproducible assessment of risks associated with realistic concentrations of different classes of antibiotics, resistance determinants, and mobile genetic elements applied to soil with organic fertilizers such as manure or digestates.

In this chapter, we will summarize recent advances, limitations, and research needs regarding approaches to quantify and evaluate the effects and risks associated with veterinary antibiotics and resistance determinants applied to soil through manure fertilization. One relevant endpoint for the environmental risk assessment (ERA) of antibiotics in the environment might represent the increase in the abundance of antibiotic-resistant bacteria and resistance genes, which can be caused by the application of resistant bacteria to the environment, the acquisition of resistance by environmental bacteria (e.g. by horizontal gene transfer), and the proliferation of indigenous resistant bacteria. For evaluation of changes in abundance of antibiotic-resistant bacteria and resistance genes, classical tools, such as quantitative real-time PCR (qPCR), on the one hand provide fast and reproducible results but are limited to known resistance gene sequences. On the other hand, rapidly advancing sequencing technologies in combination with functional screening led to the discovery of a vast diversity of novel antibiotic resistance genes and mobile genetic elements in environmental metagenomes and metamobilomes with and without human impact.[22,25] Hence, the quantification of marker genes that are widespread in the environment and affected by anthropogenic selective pressure, such as class 1 integrons, might represent a suitable approach for the evaluation of effects of antibiotics applied to soil via manure and other influencing factors. Currently, little is known about dose-response relationships and potential threshold concentrations of antibiotics applied to soil with manure.

2. Cultivation-dependent assessment of antibiotic resistance

Guidelines for ERA of pharmaceutically active compounds are available from different countries, e.g. from the European Medicines Agency or from the U.S. Food and Drug Administration. These risk assessments are typically based on traditional environmental toxicity measurements using standard tests. For example, Szatmári and colleagues[26] determined the degradation rate of doxycycline in manure-amended agricultural soil and provided ecotoxicological information regarding its effects on nitrification. In another study, Thiele-Bruhn[27] tested nine antibiotics for their effects on microbial iron(III) reduction in different soils, modeled dose-related effects, and calculated effective concentrations. However, it was demonstrated that bacteria can be affected by antibiotics even at sub-inhibitory concentrations, which not only can have considerable effects on gene expression and transcription but also can support the maintenance of resistance plasmids or select for resistant bacteria.[28–32] Furthermore, it is known that soil bacteria are a natural reservoir of antibiotic resistance determinants to both natural and synthetic antibiotics; the collection of genes that confer resistance to antibiotics is commonly referred to as the antibiotic resistome.[33–35] The application of antibiotics to soil with manure can have immediate effects on the composition of the soil bacterial community, e.g. by promoting the development, co-selection, spread, and transfer of antibiotic resistance determinants, which can indirectly affect human health if transferred to the human microbiome, e.g., by human contact with resistant bacteria in the agricultural environment or by the ingestion of vegetables from manured soil.[5] Different cultivation-dependent test methods for the assessment of resistance development and dissemination are available. One approach is to quantify bacteria resistant to a certain antibiotic within a number of isolates from an environmental sample to obtain the proportion of antibiotic-resistant bacteria within the cultivable population. These isolates can further be compared between treatments or environments by the determination of their antibiotic susceptibility, as performed by Li et al.[36] for bacteria from wastewater produced at an oxytetracycline production plant. Antibiotic-resistant bacteria can also be quantified directly using selective plating or most probable number (MPN) plates and resistance quotients can be derived from comparison with results from unselective cultivation. For example, it was observed that a high proportion of bacteria added with manure to soil microcosms were resistant to the bacteriostatic sulfonamide antibiotic sulfadiazine (SDZ) (66%) and that, up to two months after application of manure containing SDZ, the MPN counts of resistant bacteria were still significantly higher.[37] These counts might have been biased by the growth of soil bacteria with naturally reduced susceptibility to sulfonamides. However, effects of manure and SDZ on the soil bacterial community were confirmed by the quantification of sulfonamide resistance genes *sul1* and *sul2*.

Pollution-induced community tolerance (PICT) is another approach to measure changes in community tolerance after exposure to a pollutant such as an antibiotic substance.[38] For example, using Biolog® multiwell plates, Schmitt et al.[39] showed that soil treatment with the sulfonamide sulfachloropyridazine led to an increased community tolerance in bacterial soil extracts compared with the untreated control, which was enhanced upon additional soil amendment with nutrients such as pig slurry and alfalfa meal.

In another study by Brandt et al.[40], PICT was used to compare the development of tolerance to SDZ between bulk soil and nutrient-amended soil hotspots. They demonstrated that bacterial growth rates ([3H]leucine incorporation) were reduced 24 h after SDZ amendment to a concentration of 0.1 μg SDZ/g dry weight of soil, while soil respiration remained unaffected even at 100 μg SDZ/g dry weight of soil. Carbon substrate amendment *per se* led to an increased PICT response. The presence and enrichment of soil bacteria able to degrade the applied antibiotics might also have strong impacts on the evaluation of antibiotic effects on soil bacterial communities. Tappe et al.[41] could isolate a SDZ-degrading *Microbacterium* strain from soil previously manured with slurry from SDZ-medicated pigs. Topp et al.[42] showed that sulfamethazine was rapidly mineralized in soils repeatedly treated with swine manure over a period of six years. They could also culture a sulfamethazine-degrading *Microbacterium* sp. from the soil and suggested that microbial populations repeatedly exposed to livestock manures may attenuate environmental exposure to antibiotics.

Heuer and Smalla[37] compared soil treated with manure containing SDZ with untreated soil over a two-month period. Cultivation-dependent determination of SDZ-resistant bacteria, transfer frequencies, and PCR quantification of the resistance gene *sul1* revealed a transient effect of manure alone and a synergistic effect of SDZ and manure. However, the cultivation of antibiotic-resistant bacteria from soil with the subsequent physiological and genetic characterization of the isolates is limited by the extraction efficiency from soil and their culturability, which is considered to be low.[43–45]

3. PCR-based approaches

PCR-based methods allow simple and rapid cultivation-independent detection and quantification of antibiotic resistance genes in DNA extracted directly from environmental samples such as soil or manure. Classical PCR assays can only be used to determine the presence or absence of a gene in the sample, while bacterial hosts and concentrations remain unknown. Reported detection limits for PCR depend on the extraction method used and range from 10^3 to 10^8 gene copies/genomic equivalents per gram soil and 10^3 gene copies per gram soil for hybridization with digoxigenin-labeled probes.[46–48] Depending on the primers used, additional information regarding the location of genes and their association with mobile genetic elements can be obtained. These elements including integrons, transposons, and insertion sequence common region elements can be transferred by conjugative elements among soil bacteria.[6] By amplifying, for example, the variable region of class 1 integrons from community DNA and subsequent Southern blot hybridization, Binh et al.[49] demonstrated that *aadA* gene cassettes were introduced via manure into agricultural soils. Ponce-Rivas et al.[50] used PCR to evaluate the prevalence and origin of class 1 integrons and Qnr determinants in fluoroquinolone-resistant *Escherichia coli* isolates from poultry litter. They showed that resistance determinants within *E. coli* of poultry origin are genetically diverse and suggested the need for surveillance programs focused on the detection of genetic elements related to horizontal transfer genes. Despite the fact that the majority of poultry litter is applied to agricultural land, limited data are available on the ability of antibiotic-resistant bacteria and antibiotic resistance genes to persist and/or be mobilized within agricultural soils with applied poultry litters.

In contrast to "conventional" PCR, qPCR can be used to quantify genes permitting correlations to be made between the abundance of antibiotic resistance genes and the application of selective pressure over time or to evaluate concentration-dependent associations, such as the occurrence of antibiotic resistance genes and the application of manure containing antibiotics.[5,51] Typically, besides absolute quantification, the genes are quantified relative to 16S rRNA gene copies to correct for differences in amplification efficiency between samples and differences in DNA extraction or using the $2^{-\Delta\Delta C_T}$ method to compare relative changes or fluctuations in gene concentration.[52] Heuer et al.,[53] for example, observed an accumulation of sulfonamide resistance genes *sul1* and *sul2* in soil repeatedly treated with manure containing SDZ, compared with soil treated with antibiotic-free manure. In another study, Zhu et al.[7] used high-capacity qPCR-arrays to correlate the abundance of antibiotic resistance genes with antibiotic and metal concentrations in samples from commercial swine farms in China and nearby agronomic fields to which manure-based compost had been applied. However, little is known about effects of antibiotics applied to the soil over a long period of time. Knapp et al.[54] found evidence for an increase in resistance gene abundances in soils from the Netherlands between 1940 and 2008, although this increase could not be correlated directly with manure application due to the lack of quantitative data in the historic documentation.

Besides antibiotic compounds, high concentrations of antibiotic-resistant bacteria, resistance genes, and the associated mobile genetic elements such as broad-host-range plasmids are applied to soil with manure.[5,6,55–57] Manure bacteria might not be well adapted to the soil environment, and therefore the horizontal transfer of genes from manure-associated bacteria to soil-associated bacteria plays an important role in the dissemination of antibiotic resistance.[6,58] By quantifying mobile genetic elements such as broad-host-range plasmids, their role in the spread of antibiotic resistance in the environment can be assessed. IncP-1 plasmids, for example, are known to carry genes that often code for resistance to antibiotics, heavy metals, and disinfectants such as QACs.[15] The relative abundance of plasmids of the IncP-1ε subgroup in samples from pig farms was found to be positively correlated with antibiotic usage, indicating their importance for the dissemination of antibiotic resistance genes in agricultural systems.[59] It was shown that manure exposure can further increase the transferability of antibiotic resistance genes and the permissiveness of the soil bacterial community for plasmid uptake and maintenance and therefore contributes to the spread of antibiotic resistance genes.[37,60] You et al.[61] demonstrated the persistence of antibiotic resistance genes such as the tetracycline resistance gene *tet*(L) in chicken litter-impacted soil two years after the farm ceased operation. The high prevalence of *tet*(L) was explained by a group of *tet*(L)-carrying mobilizable broad-host-range plasmids, which might have contributed to the persistence of *tet*(L) in the soil bacterial community.

However, PCR-based methods are always limited by our knowledge of resistance mechanisms, resistance gene databases, and primer specificity. Moreover, these tools rely on the quality and purity of extracted DNA, which can be influenced by the soil type and extraction protocol,[62] and the sole detection of a resistance gene does not provide evidence for its activity in the respective host. Alternatively, RNA-based assays allow the analysis of gene expression but are challenging due to the short lifetime of RNA caused by the ubiquitous prevalence of ribonucleases.[63]

4. Quantification of marker genes and plasmids

The specificity of PCR in combination with the vast diversity of antibiotic resistance genes makes the general assessment of effects of antibiotics applied with manure on the abundance of resistance genes by "conventional" PCR and qPCR methods challenging. For tetracycline resistance, for example, to date, four resistance mechanisms were identified including 47 distinct classes of efflux pumps, ribosomal protection proteins, degradation enzymes, and 16S rRNA mutations that reduce the binding affinity of the drug to the ribosome.[64] This diversity of resistance genes and mechanisms might dilute the effect of selective pressure on each single resistance gene below the limit of detection and therefore might lead to an underestimation of antibiotic effects in the environment. An alternative to the direct quantification of antibiotic resistance genes might be the usage of marker genes as a proxy for the selective pressure exerted by antibiotics.

Class 1 integrons are widespread in the environment and have been proposed as a surrogate marker for anthropogenic pollution.[17,65] Class 1 integrons are genetic elements that are able to acquire, exchange, and express genes embedded in gene cassettes; these gene cassettes can contain resistance genes for almost all antibiotic families and may also contain genes encoding disinfectant and heavy metal resistance.[65,66] Class 1 integrons are not self-transferable but are often carried by mobile genetic elements such as plasmids and transposons, which facilitate their rapid transfer and spread within bacterial communities.[67] Furthermore, they are widespread in environmental compartments, observed in pathogenic and commensal bacteria of humans and animals as well as in the clinic, where all recovered *intI1* genes had essentially identical DNA sequences pointing to a common ancestor.[17,65,66] It is estimated that up to 80% of enterobacteria in humans and farm animals carry these "clinical" class 1 integrons.[65] After the application of pig slurry containing realistic concentrations of sulfachloropyridazine and oxytetracycline to soil, quantitative PCR revealed an increased relative abundance of *intI1* integrase genes, that was still detectable 10 months after application.[68] In another study, an increased abundance of *intI1* was detected in bulk soil and rhizosphere treated with manure from difloxacin-treated pigs compared with soil treated with manure from unmedicated pigs, while no effect was observed for the quinolone resistance genes tested.[69] These results suggest that concentrations of *intI1* could be used as an indicator of the general selective pressure exerted as a result of the presence of antibiotics with a higher sensitivity than could the quantification of antibiotic resistance genes alone. However, it has to be kept in mind that, in contrast to "clinical" *intI1* genes, environmental *intI1* genes exhibit a considerable but not fully surveyed sequence diversity,[70] which might limit the universality of the designed primers and hence the precise quantitative analysis. Furthermore, Jechalke et al.[17] observed an enrichment of *intI1* genes in the rhizosphere of lettuce grown in soil that did not receive manure for at least 10 years, suggesting that also other factors such as root exudation might select for bacterial populations carrying *intI1* genes.

Additionally, antibiotic resistance genes and class 1 integrons can be co-selected by other factors such as the presence of heavy metals, QACs, or stress situations in general. For example, integrase over-expression and a concomitant increase in recombination events of gene cassettes were observed in the presence of antibiotics that lead to direct or indirect DNA damage, including the antibiotic classes of fluoroquinolones, beta-lactams, trimethoprim, and aminoglycosides.[66] Besides antibiotics, co-selection of antibiotic resistance was observed, e.g. for the heavy metals copper and zinc,[16] which are regularly found in pig manure. QACs are used as disinfectants in pig farms, hospitals, and the food-processing industry and also in household products, shampoos, and cosmetics.[71–73] Resistance against QACs is mediated by *qac* resistance genes, and particularly the *qacE* and *qacEΔ1* gene variants are frequently associated with class 1 integrons.[17] Accordingly, selection with QACs could be linked to an increase in class 1 integron incidence in bacterial isolates, and the prevalence of class 1 integrons and *qac* genes in the environment was correlated with exposure to detergents and/or antibiotic residues.[18,74] Hence, co-selection is an important factor, which can influence the abundance of not only antibiotic resistance genes but also class 1 integrons in the environment. Therefore, co-selection has to be considered when using, e.g. *intI1* as a marker gene for selection by antibiotics.

Another approach to determine the concentration of antibiotics in soil that exert a selective pressure on bacterial communities is to perform competition experiments using inocula of resistance plasmid-carrying and plasmid-free bacterial populations. In a study by Jechalke et al.[75] it was demonstrated in a microcosm experiment that SDZ introduced via manure into soil provided a fitness advantage for the population of *Acinetobacter baylyi* BD413 carrying a plasmid conferring SDZ resistance, while the plasmid conferred a fitness disadvantage without selective pressure by SDZ. The authors suggest that this approach might be used in future studies for the assessment of bioavailability of antibiotic compounds in soil.

5. Next-generation sequencing approaches

Recent advances in the development of high-throughput sequencing of DNA allow for the cultivation-independent analysis of environmental community structures and functions. By correlation with environmental parameters, these approaches can be used to unravel complex ecosystem interactions and help identify responders to a specific treatment, such as the application of antibiotics with manure. In a study by Ding et al.,[76] the effect of repeated application of manure and manure containing SDZ on the soil bacterial community was explored by barcoded pyrosequencing of 16S rRNA gene fragments. It revealed bacterial taxa that were significantly enriched or decreased compared with soil treated with manure alone. Although these changes in relative abundance of taxa were in the low percentage range, which might suggest a high sensitivity of this approach, soil bacterial communities are extremely diverse and contain a large "rare biosphere" with an enormous number of low-abundance and unique taxa, which can have important ecological roles and serve as reservoirs of genetic and functional diversity.[77]

Furthermore, bacterial phylogenetic and taxonomic information alone is only able to give indications about community functions. Besides effects on bacterial community structures, metagenomic approaches combined with bioinformatic tools can provide additional functional information, e.g. on the diversity and abundance of antibiotic resistance genes. In a holistic approach, Huang et al.[78] investigated antibiotic resistance genes in activated sludge using Illumina® high-throughput sequencing in combination with 16S rRNA gene pyrosequencing and qPCR of *tet*(A), *tet*(C), and *tet*(G) resistance genes. Effects of tetracycline treatment on the bacterial community structure in sludge were observed and potentially tetracycline-resistant bacteria were identified. Furthermore, they showed by qPCR, molecular cloning and metagenomic analysis that tetracycline treatment increased the abundance and diversity of *tet* genes but decreased the occurrence and diversity of other antibiotic resistance genes.

However, similar to the case of PCR approaches discussed above, the identification of antibiotic resistance genes is limited by sequences available in the databases, and the mere detection of a gene does not prove its functionality or activity. In addition, the characterization of the genetic context of putative antibiotic resistance genes is limited by the short read length of many novel sequencing platforms.[79] In contrast, functional metagenomic selections from environmental resistomes can be used to directly link genotypes with the respective resistance phenotypes. This culture- and sequence-independent approach allows for the identification of antibiotic resistance genes in complex metagenomes by shotgun cloning of total community DNA into an expression vector and transforming the library into an indicator host.[80] Using this approach, Forsberg et al.[22] discovered approximately 3,000 antibiotic resistance genes from agricultural and grassland soils, which were mostly novel; the average amino acid identity to their closest homologue in the NCBI database was only 61.1%, emphasizing the vast diversity of known and still unknown antibiotic resistance genes within the soil resistome. Furthermore, the authors were able to correlate the resistome composition with the soil microbial phylogenetic and taxonomic structure and found indications that bacterial community composition is the primary determinant of the antibiotic resistance gene content in soil.

By functional screening of fosmid and small-insert libraries obtained from dairy cow manure, 80 different antibiotic resistance genes were identified with deduced protein sequences, which were on average only 50–60% identical to sequences deposited in GenBank.[79] Combining functional metagenomics and PacBio sequencing, the authors could analyze the genomic context and taxonomic affiliation of the antibiotic resistance genes. They found that many of the antibiotic resistance genes were affiliated to a diverse set of phyla and were flanked by mobile genetic elements, which indicates that they can be horizontally transferred between bacterial species in the cow microbiome but probably also to the environmental microbiome when applied with manure as fertilizer.

By using a combination of PCR, qPCR, and functional metagenomics, Udikovic-Kolic et al.[8] assessed the impact that manure from cows not treated with antibiotics has on the composition and resistance profiles of soil bacterial communities. They found that a higher frequency of β-lactam-resistant bacteria existed in soil amended with manure, compared with soil treated with inorganic fertilizer, which could be attributed to an enrichment of resident soil bacteria that harbor β-lactamases. However, they suggest that the lack of mobile elements in regions flanking these resistance genes may prevent their spread from soil bacteria to clinical settings.

6. Conclusions

These examples demonstrate the complexity and diversity of the soil resistome, its transferability, associated microbial taxa, and influencing factors, making it a challenge to assess the risks associated with the application of manure containing realistic concentrations of antibiotics and resistance determinants. Holistic approaches using the combination of cultivation-dependent and -independent methods may therefore be the most promising procedure for the determination of dose-response relationships and potential threshold concentrations.

Acknowledgements

S.J. was funded by the Umweltbundesamt (FKZ 3713 63 402). We thank Ilse-Marie Jungkurth for proofreading the manuscript. The authors declare that the research was conducted in the absence of any commercial or financial relationships that could be construed as a potential conflict of interest.

Author details

Sven Jechalke[1], Kimberly L. Cook[2] and Kornelia Smalla[1]

*Address all correspondence to: Kornelia.smalla@jki.bund.de

1 Julius Kühn-Institut, Federal Research Centre for Cultivated Plants (JKI), Institute for Epidemiology and Pathogen Diagnostics, Braunschweig, Germany

2 USDA, Agricultural Research Service, Food Animal Environmental Systems Research Unit, Bowling Green, KY, USA

References

[1] Cantas L, Shah SQA, Cavaco LM, Manaia C, Walsh F, Popowska M, Garelick H, Bürgmann H, Sørum H. 2013. A brief multi-disciplinary review on antimicrobial resistance in medicine and its linkage to the global environmental microbiota. *Front Microbiol* 4: 96.

[2] Stockwell VO, Duffy B. 2012. Use of antibiotics in plant agriculture. *OIE Revue Scientifique et Technique* 31: 199–210.

[3] Smith DL, Harris AD, Johnson JA, Silbergeld EK, Morris JG. 2002. Animal antibiotic use has an early but important impact on the emergence of antibiotic resistance in human commensal bacteria. *Proc Natl Acad Sci U S A* 99: 6434–6439.

[4] Du LF, Liu WK. 2012. Occurrence, fate, and ecotoxicity of antibiotics in agro-ecosystems. A review. *Agron Sustain Dev* 32: 309–327.

[5] Jechalke S, Heuer H, Siemens J, Amelung W, Smalla K. 2014. Fate and effects of veterinary antibiotics in soil. *Trends Microbiol* 22: 536–545.

[6] Heuer H, Schmitt H, Smalla K. 2011. Antibiotic resistance gene spread due to manure application on agricultural fields. *Curr Opin Microbiol* 14: 236–243.

[7] Zhu Y-G, Johnson TA, Su J-Q, Qiao M, Guo G-X, Stedtfeld RD, Hashsham SA, Tiedje JM. 2013. Diverse and abundant antibiotic resistance genes in Chinese swine farms. *Proc Natl Acad Sci U S A* 110(9): 3435–3440.

[8] Udikovic-Kolic N, Wichmann F, Broderick NA, Handelsman J. 2014. Bloom of resident antibiotic-resistant bacteria in soil following manure fertilization. *Proc Natl Acad Sci U S A* 111: 15202–15207.

[9] Forsberg KJ, Reyes A, Wang B, Selleck EM, Sommer MOA, Dantas G. 2012. The shared antibiotic resistome of soil bacteria and human pathogens. *Science* 337: 1107–1111.

[10] Yang J, Wang C, Shu C, Liu L, Geng JN, Hu SN, Feng J. 2013. Marine sediment bacteria harbor antibiotic resistance genes highly similar to those found in human pathogens. *Microb Ecol* 65: 975–981.

[11] Heuer H, Kopmann C, Binh CTT, Top EM, Smalla K. 2009. Spreading antibiotic resistance through spread manure: characteristics of a novel plasmid type with low %G plus C content. *Environ Microbiol* 11: 937–949.

[12] Perry JA, Wright GD. 2013. The antibiotic resistance "mobilome": searching for the link between environment and clinic. *Front Microbiol* 4: 138.

[13] Casey JA, Curriero FC, Cosgrove SE, Nachman KE, Schwartz BS. 2013. High-density livestock operations, crop field application of manure, and risk of community-associated methicillin-resistant *Staphylococcus aureus* infection in Pennsylvania. *JAMA Intern Med* 173: 1980–1990.

[14] Heuer H, Smalla K. 2012. Plasmids foster diversification and adaptation of bacterial populations in soil. *FEMS Microbiol Rev* 36: 1083–1104.

[15] Popowska M, Krawczyk-Balska A. 2013. Broad-host-range IncP-1 plasmids and their resistance potential. *Front Microbiol* 4: 44.

[16] Hölzel CS, Müller C, Harms KS, Mikolajewski S, Schäfer S, Schwaiger K, Bauer J. 2012. Heavy metals in liquid pig manure in light of bacterial antimicrobial resistance. *Environ Res* 113: 21–27.

[17] Jechalke S, Schreiter S, Wolters B, Dealtry S, Heuer H, Smalla K. 2014. Widespread dissemination of class 1 integron components in soils and related ecosystems as revealed by cultivation-independent analysis. *Front Microbiol* 4: 420.

[18] Gaze WH, Zhang LH, Abdouslam NA, Hawkey PM, Calvo-Bado L, Royle J, Brown H, Davis S, Kay P, Boxall ABA, Wellington EMH. 2011. Impacts of anthropogenic activity on the ecology of class 1 integrons and integron-associated genes in the environment. *ISME J* 5: 1253–1261.

[19] World Health Organization. 2014. Antimicrobial Resistance: Global Report on Surveillance. Geneva, Switzerland: WHO.ISBN 978 92 4 156474 8, www.who.int.

[20] Ashbolt NJ, Amézquita A, Backhaus T, Borriello P, Brandt KK, Collignon P, Coors A, Finley R, Gaze WH, Heberer T, Lawrence JR, Larsson DG, McEwen SA, Ryan JJ, Schönfeld J, Silley P, Snape JR, Van den Eede C, Topp E. 2013. Human Health Risk Assessment (HHRA) for environmental development and transfer of antibiotic resistance. *Environ Health Perspect* 121: 993–1001.

[21] Durso LM, Cook KL. 2014. Impacts of antibiotic use in agriculture: what are the benefits and risks? *Curr Opin Microbiol* 19: 37–44.

[22] Forsberg KJ, Patel S, Gibson MK, Lauber CL, Knight R, Fierer N, Dantas G. 2014. Bacterial phylogeny structures soil resistomes across habitats. *Nature* 509: 612–616.

[23] USEPA. 2013. Literature review of contaminants in livestock and poultry manure and implications for water quality. *Washington, DC: US Environmental Protection Agency EPA 820-R-13-002*.

[24] You Y, Silbergeld EK. 2014. Learning from agriculture: understanding low-dose antimicrobials as drivers of resistome expansion. *Front Microbiol* 5: 284.

[25] Norman A, Riber L, Luo WT, Li LL, Hansen LH, Sørensen SJ. 2014. An improved method for including upper size range plasmids in metamobilomes. *Plos One* 9 doi: 10.1371/journal.pone.0104405.

[26] Szatmári I, Barcza T, Körmöczy PS, Laczay P. 2012. Ecotoxicological assessment of doxycycline in soil. *J Environ Sci Health Part B-Pestic Contam Agric Wastes* 47: 129–135.

[27] Thiele-Bruhn S. 2005. Microbial inhibition by pharmaceutical antibiotics in different soils – dose–response relations determined with the iron(III) reduction test. *Environ Toxicol Chem* 24: 869–876.

[28] Davies J, Spiegelman GB, Yim G. 2006. The world of subinhibitory antibiotic concentrations. *Curr Opin Microbiol* 9: 445–453.

[29] Gullberg E, Cao S, Berg OG, Ilbäck C, Sandegren L, Hughes D, Andersson DI. 2011. Selection of resistant bacteria at very low antibiotic concentrations. *PLoS Pathog* 7: e1002158.

[30] Gullberg E, Albrecht LM, Karlsson C, Sandegren L, Andersson DI. 2014. Selection of a multidrug resistance plasmid by sublethal levels of antibiotics and heavy metals. *mBio* 5 doi: 10.1128/mBio.01918-14.

[31] Bernier SP, Surette MG. 2013. Concentration-dependent activity of antibiotics in natural environments. *Front Microbiol* 4: 20.

[32] Andersson DI, Hughes D. 2012. Evolution of antibiotic resistance at non-lethal drug concentrations. *Drug Resist Update* 15: 162–172.

[33] D'Costa VM, McGrann KM, Hughes DW, Wright GD. 2006. Sampling the antibiotic resistome. *Science* 311: 374–377.

[34] D'Costa VM, King CE, Kalan L, Morar M, Sung WWL, Schwarz C, Froese D, Zazula G, Calmels F, Debruyne R, Golding GB, Poinar HN, Wright GD. 2011. Antibiotic resistance is ancient. *Nature* 477: 457–461.

[35] Wright GD. 2007. The antibiotic resistome: the nexus of chemical and genetic diversity. *Nat Rev Micro* 5: 175–186.

[36] Li D, Yu T, Zhang Y, Yang M, Li Z, Liu M, Qi R. 2010. Antibiotic resistance characteristics of environmental bacteria from an oxytetracycline production wastewater treatment plant and the receiving river. *Appl Environ Microbiol* 76: 3444–3451.

[37] Heuer H, Smalla K. 2007. Manure and sulfadiazine synergistically increased bacterial antibiotic resistance in soil over at least two months. *Environ Microbiol* 9: 657–666.

[38] Boivin MEY, Breure AM, Posthuma L, Rutgers M. 2002. Determination of field effects of contaminants – significance of pollution-induced community tolerance. *Hum Ecol Risk Assess* 8: 1035–1055.

[39] Schmitt H, Haapakangas H, van Beelen P. 2005. Effects of antibiotics on soil microorganisms: time and nutrients influence pollution-induced community tolerance. *Soil Biol Biochem* 37: 1882–1892.

[40] Brandt KK, Sjøholm OR, Krogh KA, Halling-Sørensen B, Nybroe O. 2009. Increased pollution-induced bacterial community tolerance to sulfadiazine in soil hotspots amended with artificial root exudates. *Environ Sci Technol* 43: 2963–2968.

[41] Tappe W, Herbst M, Hofmann D, Koeppchen S, Kummer S, Thiele B, Groeneweg J. 2013. Degradation of sulfadiazine by *Microbacterium lacus* strain SDZm4 isolated from lysimeters previously manured with slurry from sulfadiazine medicated pigs. *Appl Environ Microbiol* 79: 2572–2577.

[42] Topp E, Chapman R, Devers-Lamrani M, Hartmann A, Marti R, Martin-Laurent F, Sabourin L, Scott A, Sumarah M. 2013. Accelerated biodegradation of veterinary antibiotics in agricultural soil following long-term exposure, and isolation of a sulfamethazine-degrading *Microbacterium* sp. *J Environ Qual* 42: 173–178.

[43] Staley JT, Konopka A. 1985. Measurement of *in situ* activities of nonphotosynthetic microorganisms in aquatic and terrestrial habitats. *Annu Rev Microbiol*. 39: 321–346.

[44] Stewart EJ. 2012. Growing unculturable bacteria. *J Bacteriol* 194: 4151–4160.

[45] Puspita ID, Kamagata Y, Tanaka M, Asano K, Nakatsu CH. 2012. Are uncultivated bacteria really uncultivable? *Microb Environ/JSME* 27: 356–366.

[46] Smalla K, van Overbeek LS, Pukall R, van Elsas JD. 1993. Prevalence of *npt*II and Tn*5* in kanamycin-resistant bacteria from different environments. *FEMS Microbiol Ecol* 13: 47-58.

[47] Pontiroli A, Travis ER, Sweeney FP, Porter D, Gaze WH, Mason S, Hibberd V, Holden J, Courtenay O, Wellington EMH. 2011. Pathogen quantitation in complex matrices: a multi-operator comparison of DNA extraction methods with a novel assessment of PCR inhibition. *PLoS ONE* 6: e17916.

[48] Hendrickx B, Junca H, Vosahlova J, Lindner A, Rüegg I, Bucheli-Witschel M, Faber F, Egli T, Mau M, Schlömann M, Brennerova M, Brenner V, Pieper DH, Top EM, Dejonghe W, Bastiaens L, Springael D. 2006. Alternative primer sets for PCR detection of genotypes involved in bacterial aerobic BTEX degradation: distribution of the genes in BTEX degrading isolates and in subsurface soils of a BTEX contaminated industrial site. *J Microbiol Methods* 64: 250–265.

[49] Binh CTT, Heuer H, Kaupenjohann M, Smalla K. 2009. Diverse *aadA* gene cassettes on class 1 integrons introduced into soil via spread manure. *Res Microbiol* 160: 427–433.

[50] Ponce-Rivas E, Munoz-Marquez ME, Khan AA. 2012. Identification and molecular characterization of class 1 integrons in multiresistant *Escherichia coli* isolates from poultry litter. *Appl Environ Microbiol* 78: 5444–5447.

[51] Walsh F, Ingenfeld A, Zampicolli M, Hilber-Bodmer M, Frey JE, Duffy B. 2011. Real-time PCR methods for quantitative monitoring of streptomycin and tetracycline resistance genes in agricultural ecosystems. *J Microbiol Methods* 86: 150–155.

[52] Livak KJ, Schmittgen TD. 2001. Analysis of relative gene expression data using real-time quantitative PCR and the 2(-Delta Delta C(T)) Method. *Methods* 25: 402–408.

[53] Heuer H, Solehati Q, Zimmerling U, Kleineidam K, Schloter M, Müller T, Focks A, Thiele-Bruhn S, Smalla K. 2011. Accumulation of sulfonamide resistance genes in arable soils due to repeated application of manure containing sulfadiazine. *Appl Environ Microbiol* 77: 2527–2530.

[54] Knapp CW, Dolfing J, Ehlert PAI, Graham DW. 2010. Evidence of increasing antibiotic resistance gene abundances in archived soils since 1940. *Environ Sci Technol* 44: 580–587.

[55] Kyselková M, Jirout J, Chroňáková A, Vrchotová N, Bradley R, Schmitt H, Elhottová D. 2013. Cow excrements enhance the occurrence of tetracycline resistance genes in soil regardless of their oxytetracycline content. *Chemosphere* 93: 2413–2418.

[56] Marti R, Tien Y-C, Murray R, Scott A, Sabourin L, Topp E. 2014. Safely coupling livestock and crop production systems: how rapidly do antibiotic resistance genes dissipate in soil following a commercial application of swine or dairy manure? *Appl Environ Microbiol* 80: 3258–3265.

[57] Binh CTT, Heuer H, Kaupenjohann M, Smalla K. 2008. Piggery manure used for soil fertilization is a reservoir for transferable antibiotic resistance plasmids. *FEMS Microbiol Ecol* 66: 25–37.

[58] Djordjevic SP, Stokes HW, Roy Chowdhury P. 2013. Mobile elements, zoonotic pathogens and commensal bacteria: conduits for the delivery of resistance genes into humans, production animals and soil microbiotia. *Front Microbiol* 4: 86.

[59] Heuer H, Binh CTT, Jechalke S, Kopmann C, Zimmerling U, Krögerrecklenfort E, Ledger T, González B, Top EM, Smalla K. 2012. IncP-1ε plasmids are important vectors of antibiotic resistance genes in agricultural systems: diversification driven by class 1 integron gene cassettes. *Front Microbiol* 3: 2.

[60] Musovic S, Klümper U, Dechesne A, Magid J, Smets BF. 2014. Long-term manure exposure increases soil bacterial community potential for plasmid uptake. *Environ Microbiol Rep* 6: 125–130.

[61] You Y, Hilpert M, Ward MJ. 2012. Detection of a common and persistent *tet*(L)-carrying plasmid in chicken-waste-impacted farm soil. *Appl Environ Microbiol* 78: 3203–3213.

[62] Frostegård A, Courtois S, Ramisse V, Clerc S, Bernillon D, Le Gall F, Jeannin P, Nesme X, Simonet P. 1999. Quantification of bias related to the extraction of DNA directly from soils. *Appl Environ Microbiol* 65: 5409–5420.

[63] Hanna SE, Connor CJ, Wang HH. 2005. Real-time polymerase chain reaction for the food microbiologist: technologies, applications, and limitations. *Journal of Food Science* 70: R49–R53.

[64] Nguyen F, Starosta AL, Arenz S, Sohmen D, Donhofer A, Wilson DN. 2014. Tetracycline antibiotics and resistance mechanisms. *Biol Chem* 395: 559–575.

[65] Gillings MR, Gaze WH, Pruden A, Smalla K, Tiedje JM, Zhu Y-G. 2014. Using the class 1 integron-integrase gene as a proxy for anthropogenic pollution. *ISME J* doi: 10.1038/ismej.2014.1226.

[66] Stalder T, Barraud O, Casellas M, Dagot C, Ploy M-C. 2012. Integron involvement in environmental spread of antibiotic resistance. *Front Microbiol* 3: 119. doi: 110.3389/fmicb.2012.00119.

[67] Gillings MR. 2014. Integrons: past, present, and future. *Microbiol Mol Biol Rev* 78: 257–277.

[68] Byrne-Bailey KG, Gaze WH, Zhang L, Kay P, Boxall A, Hawkey PM, Wellington EMH. 2011. Integron prevalence and diversity in manured soil. *Appl Environ Microbiol* 77: 684–687.

[69] Jechalke S, Focks A, Rosendahl I, Groeneweg J, Siemens J, Heuer H, Smalla K. 2013. Structural and functional response of the soil bacterial community to application of manure from difloxacin-treated pigs. *FEMS Microbiol Ecol* 87: 78–88.

[70] Gillings MR, Krishnan S, Worden PJ, Hardwick SA. 2008. Recovery of diverse genes for class 1 integron-integrases from environmental DNA samples. *FEMS Microbiol Lett* 287: 56–62.

[71] Preller L, Heederik D, Boleij JS, Vogelzang PF, Tielen MJ. 1995. Lung function and chronic respiratory symptoms of pig farmers: focus on exposure to endotoxins and ammonia and use of disinfectants. *Occup Environ Med* 52: 654–660.

[72] Buffet-Bataillon S, Tattevin P, Bonnaure-Mallet M, Jolivet-Gougeon A. 2012. Emergence of resistance to antibacterial agents: the role of quaternary ammonium compounds—a critical review. *Int J Antimicrob Agents* 39: 381–389.

[73] Holah JT, Taylor JH, Dawson DJ, Hall KE. 2002. Biocide use in the food industry and the disinfectant resistance of persistent strains of *Listeria monocytogenes* and *Escherichia coli. Symposium series (Society for Applied Microbiology)* 31: 111S–120S.

[74] Gaze WH, Abdouslam N, Hawkey PM, Wellington EMH. 2005. Incidence of class 1 integrons in a quaternary ammonium compound-polluted environment. *Antimicrob Agents Chemother* 49: 1802–1807.

[75] Jechalke S, Kopmann C, Richter M, Moenickes S, Heuer H, Smalla K. 2013. Plasmid-mediated fitness advantage of *Acinetobacter baylyi* in sulfadiazine-polluted soil. *FEMS Microbiol Lett* 348: 127–132.

[76] Ding GC, Radl V, Hai B, Jechalke S, Heuer H, Smalla K, Schloter M. 2014. Dynamics of soil bacterial communities in response to repeated application of manure containing sulfadiazine. *PLoS ONE* 9: e92958.

[77] Lynch MDJ, Neufeld JD. 2015. Ecology and exploration of the rare biosphere. *Nat Rev Micro* 13: 217–229.

[78] Huang K, Tang J, Zhang XX, Xu K, Ren H. 2014. A comprehensive insight into tetracycline resistant bacteria and antibiotic resistance genes in activated sludge using next-generation sequencing. *Int J Mol Sci* 15: 10083–10100.

[79] Wichmann F, Udikovic-Kolic N, Andrew S, Handelsman J. 2014. Diverse antibiotic resistance genes in dairy cow manure. *Mbio* 5: e01017–01013.

[80] Pehrsson EC, Forsberg KJ, Gibson MK, Ahmadi S, Dantas G. 2013. Novel resistance functions uncovered using functional metagenomic investigations of resistance reservoirs. *Front Microbiol* 4: 145.

Section 2

Antimicrobial Resistance: Impact on Humans

Chapter 3

Antimicrobial Susceptibility of Enterococcal Species Isolated from Italian Dogs

Maria Cristina Ossiprandi and Laura Zerbini

Additional information is available at the end of the chapter

http://dx.doi.org/10.5772/61778

Abstract

Monitoring planes of the occurrence of antimicrobial resistance among bacteria isolated from both animals and humans should be considered essential and strategic for preserving not only human health but also animal welfare (well-being). Moreover, the use of antimicrobial in companion animals (pets) received little attention and is not currently regulated in comparison with what happens in livestock; for this reason, the prevalence of antibiotic resistance in 165 different *Enterococcus* strains isolated from dogs (subjected to previous antibiotic treatment(s) or not) was determined. For each strain, the minimum inhibitory concentration (MIC) against 9 different antibiotics was assessed. While all isolated strains were susceptible to vancomycin, high resistance frequency toward erythromycin, rifampicin, enrofloxacin, and tetracycline was detected. *Enterococcus faecium* strains isolated from the previously treated dogs demonstrated more resistance to tetracycline compared to the control ones. Although canine enterococci showed a high degree of antibiotic resistance, they were susceptible to vancomycin, and for this reason, the hypothetical contamination of vancomycin-resistant enterococcal strains in dogs is still considered to be minimal in Italy.

Keywords: *Enterococcus*, antimicrobial susceptibility, dogs

1. Introduction

Multidrug resistance is an emerging problem in human pathogens, including zoonotic pathogens [1, 2]. Antimicrobial agents are routinely used to treat and prevent diseases in human and veterinary practices. The overuse and misuse of antibiotics provides tremendous selection, perhaps contributing spread of resistant clones, and acquisition of resistance determinants from resistant bacteria [3].

INTECH
open science | open minds

© 2015 The Author(s). Licensee InTech. This chapter is distributed under the terms of the Creative Commons Attribution License (http://creativecommons.org/licenses/by/3.0), which permits unrestricted use, distribution, and reproduction in any medium, provided the original work is properly cited.

The problem of antimicrobial resistance has been declared to be one of the top concerns of the US Centers for Disease Control (CDC) [4].

In the United States, the annual healthcare cost associated with the treatment of antibiotic-resistant infections exceeds $4 billion/year [5].

This economic burden is associated with increased severity of illness due to treatment failure and long-term hospitalization. Longer hospital stays caused increased healthcare costs and more exposure to antibiotics. This has increased the severity of illness, and mortality rate is also high.

Inappropriate use of antibiotics for therapeutic and prophylactic purposes is considered a significant contributor to the emergence of antibiotic resistance in zoonotic pathogens [6] such as MRSA (methicillin-resistant *Staphylococcus aureus*), VRE (vancomycin-resistant enterococci), and extended-spectrum β-lactamase-producing *Escherichia coli*.

Commensal bacteria have become reservoirs of antibiotic resistance genes [7]. Studies [8–10] revealed a high frequency of antibiotic resistance among the fecal microbiota in humans. Further, commensals can act as a source of horizontal transfer of resistance genes to pathogens. Similarly, clonal spread [11, 12] and the transfer of resistant genes from animal bacteria to human bacteria [12] is a concern associated with antimicrobial resistance among commensal bacteria.

Resistance gene transfer between commensals and pathogens depends on several factors such as total number of donors and recipients, nutrition, selective pressure, and transfer mechanisms. The gut gene pool is large, harboring diverse population of microbes and thus providing a suitable environment for antibiotic resistance gene transfer [7]. The level of resistance among gut commensals such as *Enterococcus* spp. is considered a good indicator of antibiotic resistance [13].

A major factor associated with the dissemination of resistant determinants is selection pressure exerted by the use of antibiotics, selecting resistant bacteria by killing the susceptible ones. The removal of selection pressure will not eliminate the resistance genes from this bacterial population [14]. This increase in the fitness cost in the absence of any antibiotic selection pressure allows rapid spread of antimicrobial-resistant strains by replacing the susceptible ones [15].

Besides selective pressure by the antibiotics, there are other factors, such as "stress in animal," that can play a role in the prevalence of resistant bacteria in the gut [16–18]. All bacteria including commensals obligate, or opportunistic pathogens within the host are subjected to stressful conditions. For example, enteric bacteria have to overcome the effects of gastric acid (with varying pH depending on the diet of the individual), bile and organic acids, competing gut commensals (for binding the receptor sites and for nutrition), and host immune responses. Animals subjected to stressors such as infection, transportation, and change in the environment can release stress hormones via the enteric nervous system. Evidence indicates that these stress hormones enhance the bacterial growth and the expression of virulence determinants in enteric pathogens [19, 20] and affect intestinal functions such as decreasing gastric acidity [21].

During the recent decades, enterococci have gained considerable attention among public health officials because of their increasing antimicrobial resistance and as important nosocomial pathogens.

Enterococci are a part of the normal microbial flora in the gastrointestinal tracts of humans, animals, and birds. The major enterococcal species include *Enterococcus faecalis*, *Enterococcus faecium*, and *Enterococcus durans*. Enterococci do not cause illness in healthy humans or animals. However, they have recently been recognized as opportunistic nosocomial pathogens that cause infections of the urinary tract (UTI) and central nervous system and lead to endocarditis and bacteremia. In addition, enterococci can rapidly acquire antimicrobial resistance through mutations or acquisition of plasmids and transposons that contain foreign genetic material, including vancomycin resistance genes [22].

In recent years, the appearance of vancomycin-resistant enterococci (VRE) has caused serious problems both in humans and in veterinary medicine [23].

Vancomycin is an antibiotic of last resort in the treatment of Gram-positive bacterial infections including enterococcal infections. The emergence of vancomycin-resistant enterococcal strains and the risk of transmission of resistance genes to the susceptible bacteria pose a serious risk to public health [24]. The presence of VRE in clinical patients results in a 20% increase in treatment failure, and mortality is also increased from 27 to 52% [25, 26].

The contribution of enterococci to the problem of antimicrobial resistance is associated with its ability to pass the resistance determinants to other bacteria of the same species or different species by the process of conjugation. Thus, resistance gene transfer to pathogenic species and emergence of new type of resistance is a serious concern associated with these bacteria. Genome sequences have revealed that one-fourth of the total genome of *E. faecalis* V583 is composed of mobile genetic elements [27]. About three to five co-resident plasmids are commonly found in clinical isolates [28, 29].

VanA, *VanB*, and *VanC* clusters determine enterococcal resistance toward glycopeptides, but the genotype *VanA* corresponds to the prevailing in terms of importance under epidemiological point of view. In fact, *VanA* genotype represents the predominant resistant one characterized by the ability to obtain inducible resistance to both teicoplanin and vancomycin. The *VanB* cluster determines inducible resistance to various levels of vancomycin, and the strains carrying it show susceptibility toward teicoplanin due to the fact that this antibiotic does not act as an inducer. The *VanC* genotype supports resistance to chromosomally encoded glycopeptide and constitutively/naturally expressed resistance to low levels of vancomycin but susceptibility toward teicoplanin. Intrinsic resistance has been recognized for *E. gallinarum*, *E. flavescens*, and *E. casseliflavus*. *E. faecium* strains resistant to vancomycin (VRE) have been isolated from different animal species (in particular from pigs, chicken, and cattle) as well as from meat derived from them. Various epidemiological studies suggest that animals can carry VRE in their intestinal microbiota and be the source of VRE infection in human (according to a classical zoonotic cycle). In fact, these VRE strains of animal origin can determine colonization of human guts expressing their pathogenicity by transferring their resistance genes to other human intestinal bacteria [23].

Cohabitation between household pets and humans creates advantageous conditions for transferring bacteria not only through direct contact such as by licking, petting, handling, and physical injuries but also through the intervention of domestic environment by food contamination as well as furnishing and so on.

Children represent the category most at risk because of their behavioral habits: close physical contact with dogs and cats but with environment eventually contaminated by the pets themselves (such as floor, toys, and carpets). It is important to remember that horizontal resistance gene transfer may occur in the opposite direction to bacterial transmission. In fact, sometimes, human bacteria that transmitted to pets can acquire resistance genes from animal microbiota and can be selected as a consequence of antimicrobial treatment occurred in these animals. Anyway, even in the case of human-to-household animal transmission, pets contribute to amplify and propagate acquired resistant bacteria through fecal shedding both in environment and in humans [30].

While there are several studies confirming the presence of VRE strains in livestock, few reports focus on the VRE colonization in household animals although VRE have been isolated from canine [31, 32] and feline gut [32] and direct contact with such animal species was considered as frequent infection source for humans [33].

A relatively high occurrence (7–23%) of VRE, mainly *E. faecium* in dogs living in urban areas, has also been reported in Europe [34].

Regular monitoring of the level of resistance in pathogens and in indicator bacteria of the normal flora, such as fecal *E. coli* and enterococci, between both humans and animals has been recommended [35, 36]. This monitoring activity is fundamental [37], allowing to match the prevalence and evolution of resistance profiles and possibly to identify resistant bacteria transferring from animals to humans and vice versa.

Thus, the aim of this study was, on the one hand, to determine the phenotypic resistance patterns in gastrointestinal enterococci in dog (with particular attention to vancomycin) and, on the other hand, to investigate whether enterococci belonging to the normal gut show more resistance in dogs that have been treated with antimicrobial therapy compared with non-treated ones.

2. Materials and methods

Ninety-nine dogs aged more than 6 months, randomly selected among those treated at the Didactic Veterinary Hospital of the Department of Veterinary Sciences in Parma (northern Italy), were collected from rectal swabs during the years 2005 and 2006.

The pets included in this research are dogs living in households located in Parma and its province. They followed a diet based on commercial products and were periodically vaccinated and treated for parasites.

In particular, fifty-six dogs had received, at least, one antimicrobial treatment over the six months preceding the survey, while the last treatment must have been made at least fourteen days before the collection of the samples.

As a whole, the dogs received 111 therapy cycles (having several subjects received two or more treatments). The formulation corresponding to amoxicillin–clavulanic acid corresponded to the most frequent (26.1%) antibiotics administered, while cephalosporins corresponded to approximately 20% of all the administered treatments; enrofloxacin and doxycycline accounted for about 15%.

The remaining 43 control dogs received no antimicrobial treatment since birth or during the preceding 12 months.

2.1. Bacteriological investigation

Rectal samples were, suitably, processed two hours after the collection. First, they were diluted in nutritive broth and kept at a temperature of 60°C in water bath; then, the samples were incubated in nutrient broth, opportunely enriched with NaCl 6.5%, and inoculated both on KF streptococcus agar (Difco) and on kanamycin aesculin azide agar base (Oxoid). After 24 and 48 h of incubation at 36°C, respectively, the suspicious colonies were subjected to biochemical characterization [38]. After conducting this initial screening, which led to the identification of a preliminary biochemical profile, the strains were identified contextually by the Rapid ID 32 Strept System and/or by the API 20 Strep System (both from bioMérieux).

After the identification, only a single strain for species belonging to the same dog has been introduced in the research (in those situations in which the same species had been isolated several times in the same subject).

2.2. Susceptibility assay

The minimum inhibitory concentration (MIC) values were obtained using microdilution test according to the Clinical and Laboratory Standards Institute (CLSI) guidelines [39].

In this study, the following nine antibiotics were tested: amoxicillin, ampicillin, ciprofloxacin, enrofloxacin, erythromycin, ofloxacin, rifampicin, tetracycline, and vancomycin. In order to reach final concentrations ranging between 64 and 0.0312 μg/ml, each antibiotic was twofold-diluted.

MIC breakpoint was always set on the basis of CLSI guidelines [39].

The isolate was considered "resistant" in the case in which its MIC was equal or greater than the values (expressed in μg/ml) reported for each antibiotic tested: amoxicillin, 16; ampicillin, 16; ciprofloxacin, 2; enrofloxacin, 1; erythromycin, 1; ofloxacin, 4; rifampicin, 2; tetracycline, 8; and vancomycin 8.

The type strain used to devise the identification scheme and to verify the quality control was *E. faecalis* ATCC 29212.

3. Results

The epidemiological study highlighted the presence of *Enterococcus* spp. strains in each fecal sample analyzed. During the identification phase, it was found the isolation of more than one species of *Enterococcus* in the same dog.

This situation allowed to isolate 165 strains from 99 fecal specimens subjected to analysis. In particular, the following species were identified: *E. avium*, *E. casseliflavus*, *E. durans*, *E. faecalis*, *E. faecium*, and *E. hirae*.

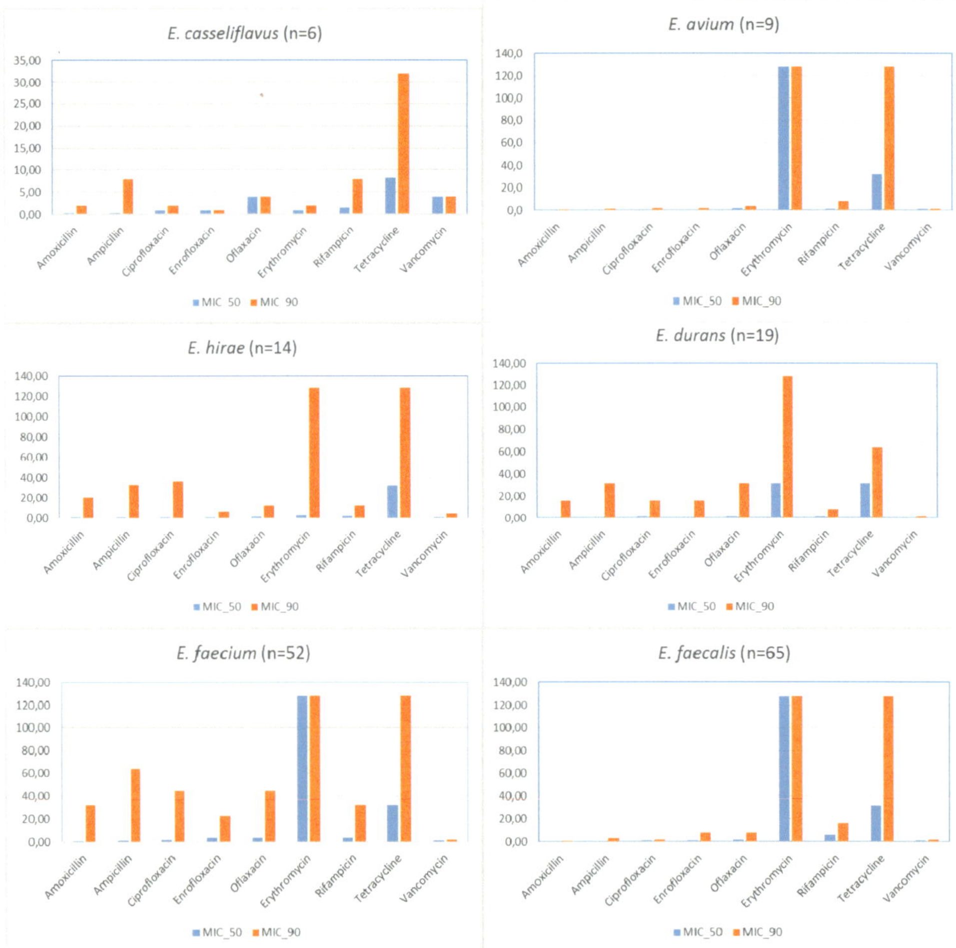

Figure 1. Results of susceptibility tests, for each species, based on MIC_{50} and MIC_{90} values [40]

Enterococcus faecalis corresponds to the prevalent species: 65 strains corresponding to 39.4% (95% CI: 32–34%), followed by *E. faecium* with 52 strains corresponding to 31.5% (95% CI: 25–39%). Together, the two above-mentioned species correspond to 70.9% of all the isolates.

Moreover, the other species isolated were 11.5% *E. durans*, 8.5% *E. hirae*, 5.5% *E. avium*, and 3.6% *E. casseliflavus*.

Results of susceptibility tests are presented in Figure 1, in which, for each species, the MIC_{50} and MIC_{90} values are summarized. These latter values represent the lowest concentration of an antimicrobial agent resulting in growth inhibition of 50% and 90% of the tested strains, respectively.

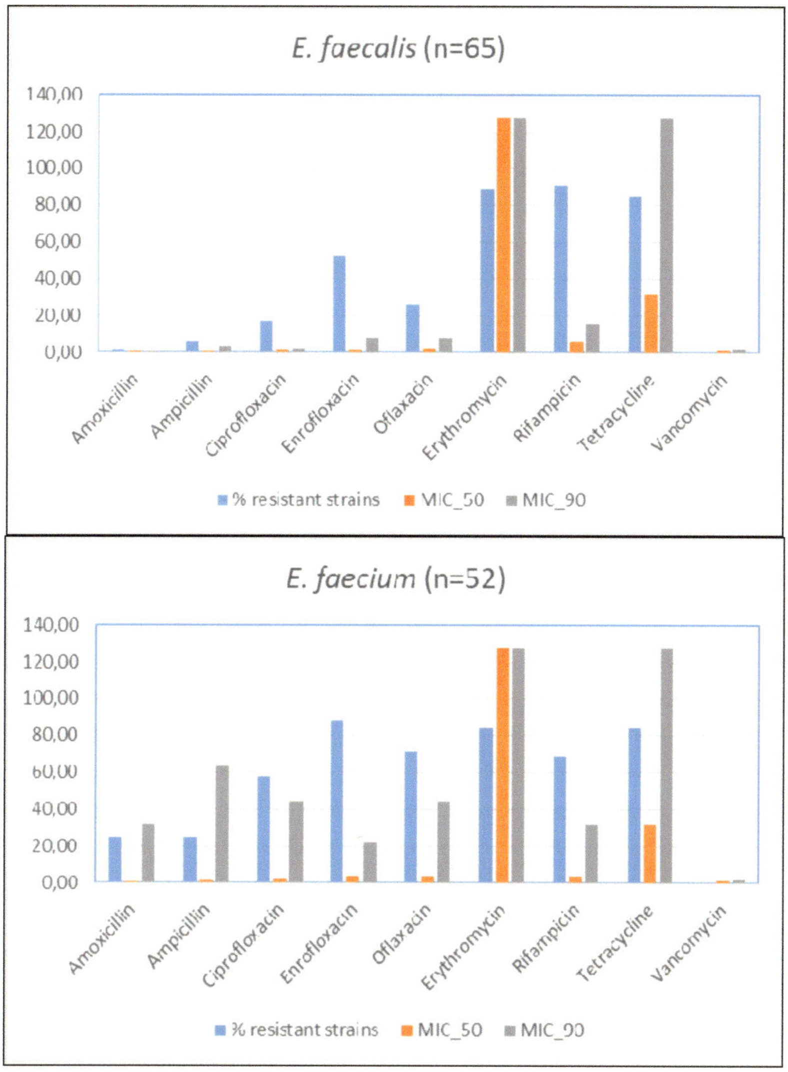

Figure 2. Cumulative percentages of multiresistance in *E. faecalis* and *E. faecium* [40]

As previously underlined, no vancomycin-resistant *Enterococcus* strains were identified and isolated; in fact, the MIC_{90} value concerning vancomycin for the two most representative

Enterococcus species above-mentioned (*faecalis* and *faecium*) was quantified as equal to 2 μg/ml. With regard to beta-lactam antibiotics, both amoxicillin and ampicillin demonstrated full action and effectiveness, representing the most effective antibiotics among the ones tested.

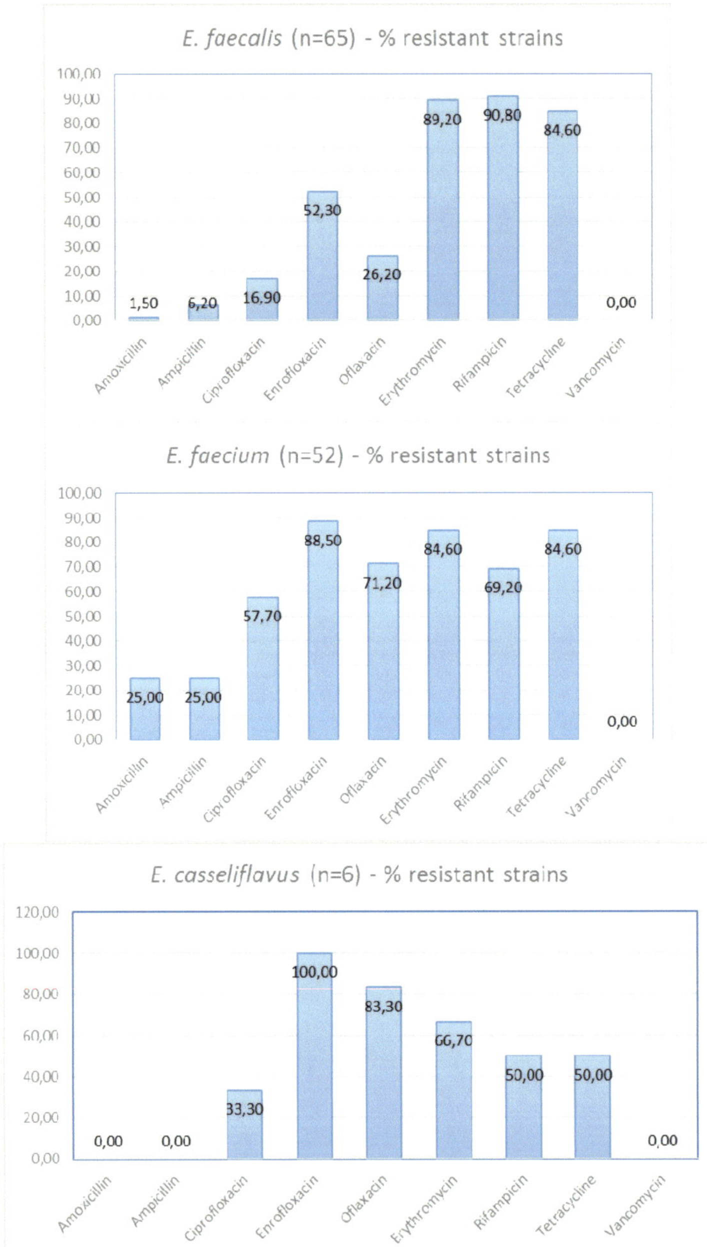

Figure 3. Resistance profile of *E. faecalis*, *E. faecium*, and *E. casseliflavus* [40]

Most strains belonging to *E. faecium* species showed quinolone resistance, while 100% of resistance to enrofloxacin was detected in *E. casseliflavus* and a high frequency of resistance (52.3%) in *E. faecalis* strains [40] (Figures 2 and 3).

The level of resistance to rifampicin, erythromycin, and tetracycline was high or very high, generally with more than 50% of strains resistant. When comparing the frequency of resistance between *E. faecalis* and *E. faecium*, we found that strains belonging to the latter species were significantly ($P < 0.05$) more resistant to the following antibiotics: amoxicillin, ampicillin, ciprofloxacin, enrofloxacin, and ofloxacin.

In Table 1, the percentages of *E. faecalis* and *E. faecium* resistant strains were reported on the basis of disaggregate data. Concerning the 117 strains evaluated, 67 (57.3%) correspond to the ones originated from dogs subjected to antibiotic treatment, while 50 isolates (42.7%) correspond to the ones from control dogs [40].

Antibiotics	***E. faecalis***		***E. faecium***	
	Treated dogs' strains (n = 36)	**Control dogs' strains (n = 29)**	**Treated dogs' strains (n = 31)**	**Control dogs' strains (n = 21)**
Amoxicillin	2.8	0.0	29.0	19.0
Ampicillin	5.6	6.9	29.0	19.0
Ciprofloxacin	13.9	24.1	67.7	42.9
Enrofloxacin	55.6	48.3	90.3	85.7
Ofloxacin	25.0	27.6	77.4	61.9
Erythromycin	94.4	79.3	90.3	81.0
Rifampicin	88.9	89.7	61.3	81.0
Tetracycline	88.9	75.9	93.5 [a]	71.4 [a]
Vancomycin	0.0	0.0	0.0	0.0

[a] $P = 0.05$. All other comparisons are not statistically significant.

Table 1. Percentages of *E. faecalis* and *E. faecium* resistant strains isolated from dogs treated and not treated with antibiotics [40]

The statistical analysis, comparing the resistance frequency in strains isolated from treated dogs and from control ones, showed a significant difference toward tetracycline ($P = 0.005$) in *E. faecium* case, with 93.5% of resistant strains isolated from treated dogs versus 71.4% from non-treated dogs. All the other comparisons were not statistically significant ($P > 0.05$).

In Figure 4, aggregate rates of multiresistance found in *E. faecalis* and in *E. faecium* are presented: it shows the cumulative percentage of strains that were resistant to one or more antibiotics tested. Over 80% of the strains belonging to both the previously mentioned species were resistant up to three antibiotics, while *E. faecalis* and *E. faecium* were, respectively, 15.4% and 41.6% resistant up to six antibiotics. Ten of the 52 *E. faecium* strains (15.4%) were resistant to all the tested antibiotics, excluding vancomycin. Multiresistance was significantly more frequent in *E. faecium* than in *E. faecalis* species [40].

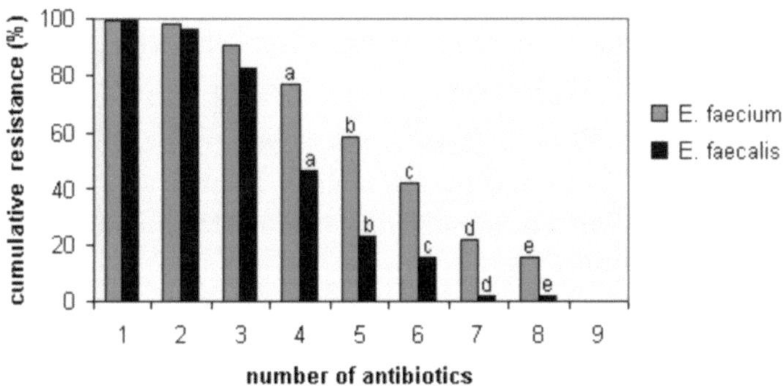

Note: Same letters indicate significantly different values ($P < 0.05$).

Figure 4. Cumulative rates of multiresistance in *E. faecalis* and *E. faecium* [40]

4. Discussion

The antibiotic resistance in bacteria, especially multidrug resistance (MDR) originating in household animals, represents a major health problem. The close contact established between pets, the dogs in this specific case, in situations of domestic coexistence clearly amplifies the possibility of bacteria transferring.

Enterococci as commensal bacteria possess natural gene transfer mechanisms and may, treacherously, spread multiple resistances. Therefore, it becomes crucial to first identify and then characterize the strains isolated from household animals [41].

Our results confirm that enterococci are constantly present in the intestine of the dog. The predominant species was shown to be *E. faecalis*, and this is in accord with De Graef et al. [42], who studied the fecal flora of dogs living in Belgium, and with Kataoka et al. [22], who analyzed fecal samples of dogs and cats.

On the contrary, Cinquepalmi et al. [34] found in southern Italy (Bari) 61.6% of *E. faecium* (45/73), 23.3% of *E. gallinarum* (17/73), and 5.5% of *E. casseliflavus* (4/73). Other species isolated (*E. raffinosus*, *E. avium*, and *E. durans*) accounted for 0.027% of the samples. *E. faecalis* was identified only in one specimen.

Studying *Enterococcus* spp. is particularly important because of their innate ability to express resistance to several antibiotics.

The research has demonstrated how *E. faecium* resistance profile versus amoxicillin, ampicillin, ciprofloxacin, enrofloxacin, and ofloxacin was significantly higher than *E. faecalis* one. This situation is confirmed by the data presented by The Surveillance Network (TSN) Database–USA [43], which shows an alarming increase in ampicillin resistance expressed by human *E. faecium* isolates.

Conversely, we found only one *E. faecalis* amoxicillin-resistant strain in the 52 strains tested; thus substantially confirming findings of De Graef et al. [44], who observed no ampicillin resistance among strains isolated from dogs.

The high resistance to erythromycin has already been observed in *E. faecalis* isolated from dogs [22], and it is probably associated with the methylation of the ribosomal target site of these antibiotics [45].

We found no vancomycin-resistant strains in the 165 samples examined, which is consistent with a number of studies on enterococci from dogs and cats [22, 34]. On the basis of this, it can be estimated that the prevalence of vancomycin-resistant strains in dog enterococcal population is <0.018 ($P = 0.05$).

Anyway, other European studies highlighted a relatively high VRE strain prevalence (mainly *E. faecium*) ranging from 7 to 23% in canine population living in contact with livestock, as well as in dogs living in urban areas. In Spain, Torres research group conducted a study on healthy animals demonstrating a higher VRE strain prevalence in household animals (23%) in comparison with swine strains (4%).

VRE occurrence has also been reported in the United States and New Zealand, countries in which the VRE presence has not been, anyhow, documented in food animals.

Dogs' VRE isolates largely contain the *VanA* resistance gene cluster and express multi resistance toward other antimicrobial categories such as tetracycline [*tet(M)* gene], macrolides [*ern(B)* gene], and aminoglycosides [*aac(6′)-aph(2′)* genes]. Therefore, even if vancomycin is generally not employed in pet veterinary practice, VRE have been considered co-selected by using such antibiotics [30].

In our study, antibiotic administration cannot be considered associated with an acquired antibiotic resistance increasing in the isolated strains analyzed, apart from tetracycline with reference to *E. faecium*. This result might be because the treatments based on tetracyclines of all our samples were carried out resorting to the use of doxycycline, a molecule that, contrary to what happens with the other tetracycline, owns a prevalently fecal excretion. This specific condition exposes the bacterial flora of the gut environment to a selective pressure for resistance.

Household dogs have long been recognized to be a potential source of zoonotic pathogens for human harboring them at intestinal level, and consequently, they have been shown to pose a significant sanitary risk for people. Humans are exposed to these pathogens through direct or indirect contact with infected dogs or their own feces, and they may also become infected after thoughtless ingestion of a zoonotic agent.

More neglected, but in any case not less important, is the fact that domestic dogs can act as the reservoir of antimicrobial-resistant agents; moreover, infections in humans and dog are often treated using similar antibiotics [30, 46].

Both the capability of non-human-origin antibiotic-resistant enterococci (e.g., sewage, raw meat, and animal feces) to colonize people and their ability to transfer resistance to human enterococci are actually not entirely known. In fact, although some researches have failed to demonstrate a relationship between antibiotic-resistant enterococci (glycopeptides included) isolated from humans and those isolated from non-human sources, some other studies have described a specific genetic relationship between *Enterococcus* strains isolated from humans and from animals (including dogs) [34].

Our study data confirmed that multiresistant enterococci (in particular, *E. faecium*) are also present in dogs even if they have never been subjected to antibiotic treatment. This result suggests that resistance transferring from dog to man should not be taken lightly.

The resistance monitoring in enterococci, which circulate between domestic animals, humans, and possibly other organisms present in the environment, and the demonstrations of similarities between resistance genes and their localization in dog and human genome could reveal many secrets of this phenomenon [44].

5. Conclusions

There are few studies that deal with the presence of microorganisms pathogenic to humans in dog feces and that address the role of these ones as a reservoir of multidrug-resistant (MDR) bacteria such as *Enterococcus*. Our study has demonstrated that in the city of Parma, northern Italy, MDR *Enterococcus* spp. were found.

Starting from the consideration that antibiotic-resistance-encoding genes can be transferred between bacteria and that actually the contact between pets and people owning domestic animals is closer than in the past, but also on the basis of our collected data, it is possible to suggest that contamination with dog feces carrying MDR microorganisms could represent a real problem for environmental and public health.

Author details

Maria Cristina Ossiprandi* and Laura Zerbini

*Address all correspondence to: mariacristina.ossiprandi@unipr.it

Department of Veterinary Medical Science, Unit of Infectious Diseases and Microbiology, Parma University, Parma, Italy

References

[1] Tenover FC, Hughes JH: The challenges of emerging infectious diseases. Journal of American Medical Association. 1996;275:300–304.

[2] Akkina JE, Hogue AT, Angulo FJ: Epidemiologic aspects, control, and importance multiple-drug resistant *Salmonella Typhimurium* DT104 in the United States. Journal of American Veterinary Medical Association. 1999;214:790–798.

[3] Levy SB: The antibiotic paradox: How the misuse of antibiotics destroys their curative powers. The New England journal of Medicine. 2002;347:1213.

[4] www.cdc.gov/ncidod/aip/research/ar.html.

[5] Stacey K: The resistance phenomenon in microbes and infectious disease vectors. 2003. Washington, DC: National Academy of Sciences.

[6] McGowan JE: Economic impact of antimicrobial resistance. Emergence Infectious Diseases. 2001;7:286–292.

[7] Marshall BM, Ochieng DJ, Levy SB: Commensals: unappreciated reservoir of antibiotic resistance. Microbe. 2009;4:231–235.

[8] Levy SB, Marshall B, Schluederberg S, Rowse D, Davis J: High frequency of antimicrobial resistance in human fecal flora. Antimicrobial Agents and Chemotherapy. 1988;32:1801–1806.

[9] Calva JJ, Sifuentes-Osornio J, Cerón C: Antimicrobial resistance in fecal flora: longitudinal community-based surveillance of children from urban Mexico. Antimicrobial Agents and Chemotherapy. 1996;40:1699–1702.

[10] Salyers AA, Gupta A, Wang Y: Human intestinal bacteria as reservoirs of antibiotic resistance genes. Trends in Microbiology. 2004;12:412–416.

[11] Kuhn I, Iversen A, Burman LG, Olsson-Liljequist B, Franklin A, Finn M, Aarestrup F, Seyfarth AM, Blanch AR, Taylor H, Caplin J, Morena MA, Dominguez L, Mollby R: Epidemiology and ecology of enterococci, with special reference to antibiotic resistant strains, in animals, humans and the environment. Example of an ongoing project within the European research programme. International Journal of Antimicrobial Agents. 2000;14:337–342.

[12] van den Bogaard AE, Stobberingh EE: Epidemiology of resistance to antibiotics. Links between animals and humans. International Journal of Antimicrobial Agents. 2000;14:327–335.

[13] Capriolo A, Busani L, Martel JL, Helmuth R: Monitoring of antibiotic resistance in bacteria of animal origin: epidemiological and microbiological methodologies. International Journal of Antimicrobial Agents. 2000;14:295–301.

[14] Salyers AA, Amabile-Cuevas CF: Why are antibiotic resistance genes so resistant to elimination? Antimicrobial Agents and Chemotherapy. 1997;41:2321–2325.

[15] Enne VI, Bennett PM, Livermore DM, Hall LM: Enhancement of host fitness by the *sul*2-coding plasmid p9123 in the absence of selective pressure. The Journal of Antimicrobial Chemotherapy. 2004;53: 958–963.

[16] Molitoris ED, Fagerberg L, Quarles CL, Krichevsky MI: Changes in the antimicrobial resistance in the faecal bacteria associated with pig transit and holding times at slaughter plants. Applied and Environmental Microbiology. 1987;53:1307–1310.

[17] Moro MH, Beran GW, Hoffman LJ, Griffith RW: Effects of cold stress on the antimicrobial drug resistance of *Escherichia coli* of the intestinal flora of swine. Letters in Applied Microbiology. 1998;27:251–254.

[18] Moro MH, Beran GW, Hoffman LJ, Griffith RW: Effects of heat stress on the antimicrobial drug resistance of *Escherichia coli* of the intestinal flora of swine. Journal of Applied Microbiology. 2000;88:836–844.

[19] Lyte M, Ernst S: Catecholamine induced growth of Gram-negative bacteria. Life Science. 1992;50:203–212.

[20] Lyte M, Arulanandam BP, Frank CD: Production of shiga like toxins by *Escherichia coli* O157:H7 can be influenced by the neuroendocrine hormones. The Journal of Laboratory and Clinical Medicine. 1996;128:392–398.

[21] Bailey MT: Psychological stress, immunity, and the effects on indigenous microflora. 2010. Microbial Endocrinology, Interkingdom Signaling in Infectious Disease and Health. New York, NY: Springer.

[22] Kataoka Y, Umino Y, Hiroki O, Kazuki H, Takuo S: Antimicrobial susceptibility of enterococcal species isolated from antibiotic-treated dogs and cats. The Journal of Veterinary Medical Science. 2014;76(10):1399–1402.

[23] Kataoka, Y, Ito C, Kawashima A, Ishii M, Yamashiro S, Harada K, Ochi H, Sawada T: Identification and antimicrobial susceptibility of Enterococci isolated from dogs and cats subjected to differing antibiotic pressures. The Journal of Veterinary Medical Science. 2013;75(6):749–753.

[24] Pearson H:"Superbug" hurdles key drug barrier. Nature. 2002;418:469.

[25] Walsh C: Molecular mechanisms that confer antibacterial drug resistance. Nature. 2000;406: 775–781.

[26] Brown DFJ, Brown NM, Cookson BD, Duckworth G, Farrington M, French GL, King L, Lewis D, Livermore DM, Macrae B, Scott GM, Williams D, Woodford N: National glycopeptides resistant enterococcal bacteremia surveillance working group report to the department of health-August 2004. Journal of Hospital Infection. 2006;62(Suppl. 1):1–27.

[27] Paulsen IT, Banerjei L, Meyers GS, Nelson KE, Seshadri R, Read TD, Fouts DE, Eisen JA, Gill SR, Heidelberg J., Tettelin H, Dodson RJ, Umayam L, Brinkac L, Beanan M, Daugherty S, DeBoy RT, Durkin S, Kolonay J, Madupu R, Nelson W, Vamathevan J, Tran B, Upton J, Hansen T, Shetty J, Khouri H, Utterback T, Radune D, Ketchum K A, Dougherty B A, Fraser CM: Role of mobile DNA in the evolution of vancomycin resistant *Enterococcus faecalis*. Science. 2003;299:2071–2074.

[28] Tomich PK, An FY, Damle SP, Clewell DB: Plasmid related transmissibility band multiple drug resistance in *Streptococcus faecalis* subsp. Zymogenes strain DS16. Antimicrobial Agents and Chemotherapy. 1979;15:828–830.

[29] Dunny G, Funk C, Adsit J: Direct stimulation of transfer of antibiotic resistance by sex pheromones in *Streptococcus faecalis*. Plasmid. 1981;6:270–278.

[30] Guardabassi L, Schwarz S, Lloyd D.H: Pet animals as reservoirs of antimicrobial-resistant bacteria. Journal of Antimicrobial Chemotherapy. 2004;54:321–332.

[31] Devriese LA, Ieven M, Goossens H, Vandamme P, Pot B, Hommez J, et al.: Presence of vancomycin resistant enterococci in farm and pet animals. Antimicrobial Agents and Chemotherapy. 1996;40:2285–2287.

[32] Van Belkun A, van den Braak N, Thomassen R, Verbrugh H, Endtz H: Vancomycin-resistant enterococci in cats and dogs. Lancet. 1996;348(9033):1038–1039.

[33] Bates J, Jordens Z, Selkon JB: Evidence for an animal origin of vancomycin-resistant enterococci. Lancet. 1993;342:490–491.

[34] Cinquepalmi V, Monno R, Fumarola L, Ventrella G, Calia C, Greco MF, de Vito D, Soleo L: Environmental contamination by dog's faeces: A public health problem? International Journal of Environmental Research and Public Health. 2013;10:72–84.

[35] Martel JL, Tardy F, Sanders P, Boisseau J: New trends in regulatory rules and surveillance of antimicrobial resistance in bacteria of animal origin. Veterinary Research. 2001;32(3-4):381–392.

[36] Van den Bogaard AE, Stobberingh EE: Epidemiology of resistance to antibiotics. Links between animals and humans. International Journal of Antimicrobial Agents. 2000;14(4):327–335.

[37] Herrero IA, Fernández-Garayzábal JF, Moreno MA, Domínguez L: Dogs should be included in surveillance programs for vancomycin-resistant Enterococci. Journal of Clinical Microbiology. 2004;42(3):1384–1385.

[38] Manero A, Blanch AR: Identification of *Enterococcus* spp. with a biochemical key. Applied and Environmental Microbiology. 1999;65(10): 4425–4430.

[39] Clinical and Laboratory Standards Institute. Performance Standards for Antimicrobial Susceptibility Testing: Fifteenth Informational Supplement. Villanova, PA: CLSI; 2005 Publication No. M100–S15.

[40] Ossiprandi MC, Bottarelli E, Cattabiani F, Bianchi E: Susceptibility to vancomycin and other antibiotics of 165 *Enterococcus* strains isolated from dogs in Italy. Comparative Immunology, Microbiology and Infectious Diseases. 2008;31:1–9.

[41] Jackson CR, Fedorka-Cray PJ, Davis JA, Barrett JB, Frye JG: Prevalence, species distribution and antimicrobial resistance of enterococci isolated from dogs and cats in the United States. Journal of Applied Microbiology. 2009;107:1269–1278.

[42] De Graef EM, Devriese LA, Baele M, Vancanneyt M, Swings J, Haesebrouck F, et al.: Identification of enterococcal, streptococcal and *Weissella* species in the faecal flora of individually owned dogs. Journal of Applied Microbiology. 2005;99(2):348–353.

[43] Huycke MM, Sahm DF, Gilmore MS: Multiple-drug resistant Enterococci: the nature of the problem and an agenda for the future. Emerging Infectious Diseases. 1998;4(2): 239–249.

[44] De Graef EM, Decostere A, Devriese LA, Haesebrouck F: Antibiotic resistance among fecal indicator bacteria from healthy individually owned and kennel dogs. Microbial Drug Resistance. 2004;10(1):65–69.

[45] Leclerq R, Courvalin P: Bacterial resistance to macrolide, lincosamide and streptogramin antibiotics by target modification. Antimicrobial Agents and Chemotherapy. 1991;35:1267–1272.

[46] Sternberg S: Antimicrobial resistance in bacteria from pets and horses. Acta Veterinaria Scandinavica. 1999;92:37–50.

Chapter 4

Review - Understanding β-lactamase Producing *Klebsiella pneumoniae*

Marisa B. De Jesus, Marthie M. Ehlers, Ricardo F. Dos Santos and Marleen M. Kock

Additional information is available at the end of the chapter

http://dx.doi.org/10.5772/61852

Abstract

Klebsiella pneumoniae is a nosocomial pathogen commonly implicated in hospital outbreaks with a propensity for antimicrobial resistance towards mainstay β-lactam antibiotics and multiple other antibiotic classes. The successful proliferation, transmission and infection of the Gram-negative bacterium can be attributed to a myriad of factors including host factors, environmental factors, virulence factors and a large repertoire of antibiotic resistance mechanisms. The poor treatment outcomes and limited treatment options are consequences of the successful pathogenesis and spread of antibiotic resistance in the increasingly common β-lactamase producing *K. pneumoniae* bacterium. The review briefly explores the biology, successful pathogenesis and antibiotic resistance of *K. pneumoniae* as well as the detection and characterisation techniques of important strains.

Keywords: *Klebsiella pneumoniae*, β-lactamases, Antibiotic resistance

1. Introduction

The evolution of the Gram-negative bacillus in an era of antibiotic use has resulted in a changed epidemiology, wherein *K. pneumoniae* now commonly occurs in healthcare facilities, such as hospitals, and is responsible for a range of serious infections involving the urinary tract, lungs, abdominal cavity, intra-vascular devices, soft tissues surgical sites and causing bacteraemia [1]. Treatment of *K. pneumoniae* infections has been complicated by the rapid and easy acquisition of antimicrobial resistance along with the unmatched development of novel antimicrobials to combat them [1–5]. Resistance determinants in *Enterobacteriaceae* are typically encoded on the chromosome, plasmids, integrons and transposons [6]. *Klebsiella pneumoniae* is an *Enterobacteriaceae* member which often displays resistance towards β-lactam antibiotics,

INTECH
open science | open minds

© 2015 The Author(s). Licensee InTech. This chapter is distributed under the terms of the Creative Commons Attribution License (http://creativecommons.org/licenses/by/3.0), which permits unrestricted use, distribution, and reproduction in any medium, provided the original work is properly cited.

particularly through β-lactamase expression of which the most important are cephalosporinases, such as extended-spectrum β-lactamases (ESBLs) and carbapenemases [6].

Several mechanisms contribute towards antimicrobial resistance and virulence in Gram-negative bacteria and may even work in concert to achieve multidrug resistance profiles [7–8]. Resistance determinants usually mediate resistance by inactivating the antimicrobial agent, modifying the antibiotic or its target and decreasing antimicrobial drug concentrations within the cell [9–11]. A common form of enzymatic inactivation of antibiotics is the acquisition and expression of β-lactamase genes within bacterial species, such as *K. pneumoniae*, which can be classified into Ambler classes A to D [12]. Extended-spectrum β-lactamases typically confer resistance towards penicillins, first-, second- and third-generation cephalosporins as well as aztreonam, but remain mostly inhibited by clavulanic acid, an inhibitor [13]. Extended-spectrum β-lactamase-producers can additionally express resistance towards other antibiotics, such as aminoglycosides and fluoroquinolones, and are typically treated with carbapenems [2,3,5,14]. The use of antibiotics, such as aminoglycosides, carbapenems, cephalosporins, fluoroquinolones as well as β-lactam/β-lactamase inhibitors, has been identified as one of the several risk factors associated with carbapenem-resistant *Enterobacteriaceae* (CRE) infection [15,16]. Treatment of CREs are often reliant on last resort antimicrobials, such as colistin, fosfomycin and/or tigecycline, which can be rendered ineffective due to antimicrobial resistance evolving or emerging [4,16–18]. The rise in carbapenemase-producers both locally and internationally poses a treatment dilemma as fewer efficacious antibiotics are available and all are threatened in light of the emergence of extensively drug-resistant (XDR) and pan-drug-resistant (PDR) Gram-negative bacteria [16]. Carbapenem resistance in *Enterobacteriaceae* has been detected worldwide at alarming frequencies, including in Africa, Asia, Europe, North America and South America [19–22]. The prevalence and geographical distribution of various *K. pneumoniae* strains differ, but a particularly important strain involved in national and international epidemics is the sequence type (ST) 258 harbouring the *K. pneumoniae* carbapenemase (KPC) [19,23–25].

Characterisation of clinically relevant *K. pneumoniae* isolates has elucidated strains implicated in both community-associated and healthcare-associated infections, of which the former has displayed a metastatic spread uncommon for enteric Gram-negative bacilli [1,15,26]. Clinical manifestations of infection and even geographical restriction of particular infections can be attributed to a myriad of factors, inclusively virulence factors and host-associated factors [26, 27]. The hypervirulent *K. pneumoniae* (hvKP) strains, variants of the "classical" *K. pneumoniae*, typically cause pyogenic liver abscesses, pneumonia, meningitis and endophthalmitis in otherwise healthy individuals [1]. "Classical" *K. pneumoniae* strains have typically exhibited a propensity for multidrug-resistance acquisition, whereas hvKP has remained largely susceptible with only a few reports of multidrug-resistant (MDR)-hvKP [1].

Once established in the hospital setting, the proliferation and spread of MDR strains can occur within and between hospitals [28]. The molecular characterisation of β-lactamases and the molecular typing of *K. pneumoniae* MDR isolates thus provide insight into current resistance profiles and possible routes of transmission. Whether by evolution of local clones through genetic determinant acquisition or introduction of successful international clones and their β-lactamases, the increase in multidrug-resistant *K. pneumoniae* isolates can be associated with poor treatment outcome [1,29,30]. The diversity and high number of resistance genes found in *K. pneumoniae* are indicative of an ever-growing resistance gene pool [31]. Future research should thus encompass deeper analysis of virulence factors implicated in the successful pathogenesis of *K. pneumoniae* working in concert with the existing β-lactamases, which attribute to its survival and proliferation within and outside its host. In addition, whole genome sequencing of important *K. pneumoniae* strains with multidrug resistance and the use of computational tools is an important next-step for elucidating gene characteristics, such as the virulence genes, through comparative genomics [32,33].

2. Epidemiology of multidrug-resistant *Klebsiella pneumoniae*

Klebsiella pneumoniae is a nosocomial pathogen commonly isolated from the intensive care unit (ICU) and implicated in hospital outbreaks, which is increasingly displaying high drug-resistant profiles through β-lactamase production, such as ESBL production and globally emerging carbapenem resistance [3,21,27,34]. The existence of β-lactamase enzymatic activity was first observed in 1940, which is prior to the implementation of penicillin for treatment [12]. The existence of the β-lactamases was therefore naturally present within environmental isolates [12,35,36].

Broad-spectrum β-lactamases initially emerged in *E. coli* during the 1960s and 1970s but rapidly spread to other bacterial species, including within the *Enterobacteriaceae* family, which led to treatment using second- and third-generation cephalosporins [11,37,38]. The first β-lactamase enzyme described in 1965 was the Temoneria (TEM)-1 enzyme and soon thereafter the sulphydryl variable (SHV)-1 β-lactamase, which can typically confer resistance to penicillins but not to cephalosporins [39]. Temoneria- and SHV-type β-lactamase derivatives described as ESBLs were soon thereafter detected and found to have activity against oxyimino-β-lactam antibiotics through minor active site modifications [14,39,40]. Resistance to oxyimino-β-lactam antibiotics was recorded briefly after (year 1982) the introduction of third-generation cephalosporins in *K. pneumoniae* and *Serratia marcescens* [41].

Hospital outbreaks of ESBL-producing bacteria, particularly *K. pneumoniae* and *E. coli*, are a threat that has existed for several years, since its first recorded outbreak in French hospitals in the 1980s [42–44]. Historically, the predominating β-lactamases encoded were of the TEM- or SHV-type, for example, in the United States of America, but a shift has occurred with the Cefotaximase-Munich (CTX-M)-type being the most commonly detected ESBL [44,45]. Worldwide distribution of ESBL-producing *Enterobacteriaceae*, especially *K. pneumoniae* and *E. coli* encoding CTX-M, has been recorded with an increase in prevalence over the years [46]. The predominating ESBL enzyme within clinical isolates mediating resistance can be geographically variable [44]. The lack of consistent studies or few studies reporting on the ESBL prevalence and genes detected in some African countries, particularly within Eastern and Western Africa, makes it difficult to determine trends in antimicrobial resistance patterns [22]. Non-ESBL-resistant phenotypes are also still present in clinical isolates and are attributed to the production of broad-spectrum β-lactamases, such as TEM-1, TEM-2 and SHV-1 [47]. Alternately, high-level resistance can be attributed to inhibitor-resistant β-lactamases, which are TEM derivatives or due to cephalosporinase production [47]. Several other ESBL variants exist [48]. The only Ambler class D ESBLs are of the OXA-type enzymes of which OXA-1 has been frequently associated with other ESBL encoding genes and OXA-2 with PER-1 ESBLs [48–50]. The result of the former OXA-1 association with other ESBLs, particularly with $bla_{\text{CTX-M}}$ genes, could be β-lactam-β-lactamase inhibitor combination resistance [49]. Infections by ESBL-producing *K. pneumoniae* ranging from urinary tract infections to complicated sepsis are preferentially treated with the carbapenem antibiotic [3–14].

Carbapenem resistance in *Enterobacteriaceae* has been detected worldwide at alarming frequencies, including in Africa, Asia, Europe, North America and South America [19–22]. The prevalence and geographical distribution of various *K. pneumoniae* strains differ, but a particularly important strain involved in national and international epidemics is the sequence type (ST) 258 harbouring the *K. pneumoniae* carbapenemases (KPC) [19,23–25]. The most important carbapenemases belong to the Ambler Class A [*K. pneumoniae* carbapenemase (KPC)], Class B [metallo-β-lactamases (MBL), such as New Delhi metallo-β-lactamases (NDM-1)] and Class D [Oxacillinases, particularly OXA-48-type carbapenemases] [6,20,25, 51,52].

3. Classification of *K. pneumoniae* isolates

Klebsiella belongs to the Phylum *Proteobacteria,* the Class *Gammaproteobacteria* and the Order *Enterobacteriales.* The genus *Klebsiella* further belongs to the *Enterobacteriaceae* family and can be subdivided into a range of species, including *Klebsiella granulomatis, K. mobilis, K. ornithinolytica, K. oxytoca, K. planticola, K. pneumoniae, K. singaporensis, K. terrigena, K. trevisanii* and *K. variicola* [53–55]. The bacterium *K. pneumoniae* can be further subdivided into *K. pneumoniae* subsp. *pneumoniae, K. pneumoniae* subsp. *ozaenae* and *K. pneumoniae* subsp. *rhinoscleromatis* (Table 2.1) [53,55,56]. *Klebsiella pneumoniae* is closely related to several other genera within the *Enterobacteriaceae* family, such as *Citrobacter, Escherichia, Enterobacter* and *Salmonella* [11,57].

A study conducted by Drancourt and collegues (2001) aimed at re-establishing and confirming the taxonomy of the genus *Klebsiella* determined the carbon assimilation patterns, 16S rDNA and β-subunit of RNA polymerase B (*rpo*B) sequences for eight *Klebsiella* species [54]. Seven of the *Klebsiella* species, namely *K. ornithinolytica, K. oxytoca, K. planticola, K. pneumoniae* subsp. *ozaenae, K. pneumoniae* subsp. *pneumoniae, K. pneumoniae* subsp. *rhinoscleromatis* and *K. terrigena,* could be distinguished by the inability of the *K. pneumoniae* subspecies to grow at 10°C or utilise L-sorbose as the sole carbon source [54]. The 16S rDNA and *rpo*B sequence analyses furthermore indicated a 98.2% to 99.7% and 99.4% to 100% similarity, respectively, between the three *K. pneumoniae* subspecies and *K. granulomatis* [54]. Sequence analysis of the *rpo*B gene is confirmatory for *K. pneumoniae* but is typically used for characterisation utilising MLST [28, 58]. *Klebsiella pneumoniae* is the most relevant and common species isolated from clinical specimens [59].

4. General characteristics of *K. pneumoniae* bacteria

Klebsiella species are ubiquitous and can occur within two broadly defined habitats, namely the environment and mucosal surfaces of mammals, including humans [59]. In the environment it can be found to exist in surface water, sewage, soil and even on plants whilst on their human host the saprophyte can be located in the nasopharynx and the intestinal tract [59]. The human skin is not conducive for the growth of *Klebsiella* species and so is merely considered to be transiently colonised [59].

Klebsiella pneumoniae presents typically as Gram-negative straight rods between 0.3 and 1.8 μm in size [60]. The non-motile bacteria are lactose-fermenting, facultative anaerobes that proliferate at 37°C and produce characteristically mucoid colonies on carbohydrate- rich media, attributed to the presence of a capsule [54,60]. Biochemical reactions can be utilised for the identification and differentiation of *Klebsiella* species [59].

4.1. Culture and metabolic characteristics

Klebsiella species are easily cultured on media suitable for *Enterobacteriaceae* bacteria, including: nutrient agar, tryptic casein soy agar, bromocresol purple lactose agar, Drigalski agar, MacConkey agar, eosin-methylene blue (EMB) agar and bromothymol blue (BTB) agar [61]. No additional growth factors are required by *K. pneumoniae,* which is capable of both fermentative and respiratory metabolism [54]. The facultative anaerobe can have a variable mucoid appearance, which may vary between different strains and be influenced by the composition of the medium used [54,61].

Useful tests in determining enterobacterial taxonomy include carbon source utilisation tests, glucose oxidation test in the presence or absence of pyrroloquinoline quinone, gluconate- and 2-ketogluconate dehydrogenase tests and tetathionate reductase and β-xylosidase tests [62]. All *Klebsiella* strains are capable of utilising L-arabinose, D-arabitol, D-cellobiose, citrate D-fructose, D-galactose, D-glucose, 2-ketogluconate, maltose, D-mannitol, D-melibiose, D-raffinose, D-trehalose and D-xylose, whilst lactose and D-sorbitol can be used as a carbon source by all strains, except *K. pneumoniae* subsp. *ozaenae* and *K. pneumoniae* subsp. *Ornithinolytica* [61]. A unique characteristic to both *K. pneumoniae* subsp. *pneumoniae* and *K. mobilis* is the ability to oxidise glucose to gluconate using glucose dehydrogenase in the absence of pyrroloquinoline quinone [61]. *Klebsiella pneumoniae* subsp. *pneumoniae* in addition possesses enzymes involved in the glycerol dissimilation pathway, namely glycerol dehydrogenase type I and 1,3-propanediol dehydrogenase, which permits fermentative growth on glycerol [32,61,63,64].

Klebsiella species are oxidase negative, catalase positive and often Voges-Proskauer test positive, with the exception of *K. pneumoniae* subsp. *ozaenae* and *K. pneumoniae* subsp. *Rhinoscleromatis* [54,61]. Most strains can hydrolyse urea, reduce nitrates without the production of H_2S gas, as well as utilise glucose and citrate as carbon sources [54]. In the case of fermentation of glucose, a gas and an acid are produced [54]. Glucose fermentation also results in the formation of acetoin and 2,3-butanediol [61].

4.2. Genomic characteristics

Klebsiella pneumoniae isolates' genome size ranges from 5.1 to 5.6 Mb with extensive genetic variation being reported among intraspecific strains due to genomic rearrangements (often as a result of chromosomal inversions, plasmids and mobile genetic elements) as well as strain-specific genes [11,65]. The nine *K. pneumoniae* subsp. *pneumoniae* whole genomes currently available on public databases [NCBI GenBank Entrez Genome database (http://www.ncbi.nlm.nih.gov/genome)] include: *K. pneumoniae* strain MGH78578, NTUH-K2044, 342, HS11286, KCTC2242, CG43, JM45, KP13 and 1084 [32,65]. In a study conducted by Kumar and colleagues (2011) where two *K. pneumoniae* strains were sequenced and compared with previously sequenced strains, 3 631 common proteins were identified and considered to be the core set of orthologous genes [11]. A comparison with the information on known biological functions of 342 *K. pneumoniae* proteins revealed that 52.11% of the protein-encoding genes were dedicated to transport and binding proteins, energy metabolism, regulatory function and cell envelope, respectively [11]. A five-gene cluster involved in anaerobic sugar metabolism that was also identified in two of the strains, namely strain 1162281 and JH1, was found to be similar to Gram-positive genera homologs [11]. In a separate study by Ramos and colleagues (2014), the Kp13 chromosome was compared to strains MGH78578, NTUH-K2044 and 342 and it was found to harbour a similar G+C content (57.5%, 57.5%, 57.7% and 57.3%, respectively) [65]. The G+C content for Kp13 was, on the other hand, lower for the six plasmids, suggestive of DNA acquired through horizontal gene transfer (HGT) [65]. At least 32 *K. pneumoniae* plasmids have been sequenced, which range in size from 3 to 270 kb [66].

Microbial pathogens are capable of modifying inherent virulence or patterns of spread through evolutionary processes, which can often be mediated by HGT [1]. The acquisition of pathogenicity islands and virulence plasmids are mechanisms by which *K. pneumoniae* may laterally transfer genes [1]. Resistance genes could also be acquired by Gram-negative bacteria through recombination, integron-mediated mobilisation of gene cassettes or transposition [67]. An example of a lateral plasmid transfer mechanism is the acquisition of a large 180 to 220 kb virulence plasmid by hypervirulent *K. pneumoniae* (hvKP) strains that are not typical in "classical" *K. pneumoniae* strains and encode virulence factors, such as the RmpA (regulator of the mucoid phenotype) and iron acquisition factors [1].

Klebsiella pneumoniae has acquired multiple resistance genes over time [67]. The common statement that antibiotic use is solely to blame for increased antibiotic resistance over time is challenged by Projan (2007), who hypothesised that the ability of a bacterium to develop resistance could be a function of genome size because larger genomes have more genetic information to draw from [68]. In support of this school of thought, smaller genomes of some bacteria appear more specialised, such as *Treponema pallidum*, whereas those with larger genomes are more environmentally adaptable and versatile, such as *K. pneumoniae* and *Acinetobacter baumannii*, thus developing multidrug resistance more easily [68]. Resistance genes acquired, particularly ESBL genes, are widely disseminated even between species, such as strains of *Escherichia coli*, *Enterobacter aerogenes*, *Proteus mirabilis* and *Pseudomonas aeruginosa* [48].

5. Virulence factors and the role in pathogenesis of *K. pneumoniae*

The significant impact of *K pneumoniae* in the clinical setting as a healthcare-associated pathogen has prompted investigation into the factors implicated in its pathogenesis [7]. The factors aiding in basic pathogenesis of *K. pneumoniae* are the fimbrial and non-fimbrial adhesins, a capsule, siderophores (particularly enterobactin), urease, lipopolysaccharide (LPS), serum resistance as well as biofilm formation [7,8,46,69,70,71]. On the other hand, enhancing factors aiding invasion include other siderophores (aerobactin and yersiniabactin), catechols receptor, mucoid factor and hypermucoviscosity [8,72].

The prerequisite to an infection is often the mucosal pathogen's ability to adhere [7,73]. *Klebsiella pneumoniae* expresses numerous fimbrial and non-fimbrial adhesins capable of recognising varied receptors, which in turn can facilitate the adherence to several target cells [7]. Fimbrial adhesins include mannose-sensitive type 1 fimbriae, type 3 fimbriae and plasmid-encoded fimbriae designated as KPF-28, while a non-fimbrial adhesin includes the CF29K factor [7,59,61,70,74,75]. The above mentioned type 1 and type 3 fimbriae are frequently detected in *K. pneumoniae* isolates, particularly mediating urinary tract infections (UTIs) and biofilm formation, respectively [8,65,75]. The expression of the various fimbriae can be both beneficial in that it may facilitate attachment or disadvantage the bacterium due to the heightened host immune response that may be triggered, thus outlying the opportunistic nature of *K. pneumoniae* [7].

Surface saccharides that have been associated with *K. pneumoniae* virulence in a human host include an LPS and capsule [69]. Capsules can play an important role outside the human host by offering some protection against desiccation in the environment or in the host by resisting complement-mediated lysis or phagocytosis and possibly having a neutralising effect against antibodies through the release of excessive capsular material [69,76,77]. At least 78 antigenically varied capsular types have been identified in *K. pneumoniae* [1,78–81] Resistance to phagocytosis was found to be higher in K1 and K2 capsular serotypes [1,82]. Particular types may also play a more significant role in virulence, such as the K2 capsule, which has frequently been isolated from clinical isolates implicated in urinary tract infections, pneumonia and bacteraemia [7,46,61,79]. The LPS is, on the other hand, a component situated in the outer membrane of bacteria and part of it forms the O-antigen of which there are only 12 differing antigens [59,61].

Finally, the growth of *K. pneumoniae in vivo* necessitates essential elemental iron for which it competes with the host by producing high-affinity extracellular ferric chelators (iron-binding molecules) [7,72]. A hypervirulent strain of *K. pneumoniae* was found to possess greater quantities of biologically active siderophores [1,72]. The genes encoding siderophores include *ent*B (enterobactin), *iut*A (aerobactin), *irp*1-*irp*2-*ybt*S-*fyu*A (yersiniabactin) and *iro*N (ferric-catecholates receptor) [72].

Virulence genes typically researched include *uge* (encoding uridine diphosphate galacturonate 4-epimerase), *wab*G (involved in the biosynthesis of the outer core lipopolysaccharide), *ure*A (related to the urease operon), *mag*A (mucoviscosity-associated gene A), *mrk*D (type 3 fimbriae adhesion), *all*S (activator of the allantoin regulon), *kfu*BC (iron-uptake system), *rpm*A (regulator of mucoid phenotype) and *fim*H (fimbrial gene encoding type 1 fimbrial adhesion) due to their role in bacterial pathogenesis [32,80,83]. The virulence of *K. pneumoniae* is further exacerbated by the additional, easy acquisition of β-lactamase encoding genes; however, successful infection is ultimately also reliant on a number of host-dependent factors [8].

6. Clinical manifestations of *K. pneumoniae* infections

Klebsiella pneumoniae is both known as a commensal bacterium found in the environment and as an important healthcare-associated pathogen involved in a myriad of infections, ranging from blood, respiratory, urinary and intra-abdominal infections, in predominantly incapacitated patients [62,73,75,80,84]. Clinical presentations of disease caused by *K. pneumoniae* are affected by the quantity and type of virulence factors expressed, whereas the resulting infections can be divided into community-associated and healthcare-associated infections [26,75].

Klebsiella pneumoniae mostly affects patients in the ICU and is an important contributor to in-hospital mortality [3]. In the clinical setting, *K. pneumoniae* is second only to *E. coli* in causing catheter-associated urinary tract infections and is an important blood stream pathogen [27,75]. On the other hand, *K. pneumoniae* is also responsible for diseases, such as community-associated pneumonia, pyogenic liver abscess, rhinoscleroma, atrophic rhinitis and less frequently meningitis, necrotising fasciitis and prostatic abscess [75,80,85–87]. Rhinoscleroma and atrophic rhinitis are specifically caused by *K. pneumoniae* subsp. *rhinoscleromatis* and *K. pneumoniae* subsp. *Ozaenae*, respectively [80]. Community-associated infections, such as pneumonia and liver abscesses, meningitis or endophthalmitis have been identified in Taiwan and South Africa [26]. *Klebsiella pneumoniae* implicated in community-associated meningitis led to mortality rates ranging from 30% to 83% in adult cases with added severe neurologic sequelae in survivors in South Africa [72]. It was also noted that bacteraemic community-associated pneumonia mediated by *K. pneumoniae* had a poorer prognosis than *Streptococcus pneumoniae* mediated bactereamia [88].

Unlike their Gram-positive counterparts, invasive infections and metastatic spread are rare for extra-intestinal Gram-negative pathogens, such as *K. pneumoniae* [72,73]. Hypervirulent strains of *K. pneumoniae* have, on the other hand, been identified and associated with community-associated liver abscesses as well as spread to bone, eyes, joints, kidneys, lungs, muscle/fascia, pleura, prostate, spleen, soft-tissue, skin and the central nervous system (CNS) [72,73]. *Klebsiella pneumoniae* is largely thought of as an opportunistic pathogen, but the emergence of hypervirulent strains over the past decade have demonstrated the capacity to infect otherwise healthy individuals [72,73].

The virulence factors expressed could contribute to the range of clinical manifestations of infections, but the geographical restriction of certain manifestations could alternately be dependent on host factors typical to that region [26,27,89]. Host factors could include the frequency of diabetes mellitus, genetic predilections, underlying prevalent diseases, alcoholism, socioeconomic determinants and the availability of quality healthcare [26,27,89,90].

7. Treatment of *K. pneumoniae* infections

Appropriate therapeutic options are often determined based on the antibacterial spectrum, convenience of use and tolerability of antimicrobials, such as third- and fourth-generation cephalosporins.[91] The factors influencing appropriate antimicrobial treatment are also dependent on local bacterial susceptibility patterns and patient risk profiles, which may ultimately determine the risk of infection with opportunistic and potentially antibiotic-resistant pathogens [92]. Multidrug-resistant bacterial strains, such as *K. pneumoniae, Pseudomonas aeruginosa* and *Acinetobacter baumannii,* present a therapeutic conundrum due to their ability to undermine treatment, whilst also reducing appropriate antibiotic options available and causing a delay in appropriate treatment due to inefficient empirical treatment [29,93].

7.1. Treatment of multidrug-resistant *K. pneumoniae* infections

The global emergence of multidrug-resistant Gram-negative bacilli is an unprecedented problem, which is exacerbated by the focus on improving existing classes of drugs instead of developing new classes of drugs with alternate targets over the past 50 years [4,5]. The rise in the rate of multidrug-resistant bacteria and the increasingly limited treatment options is exemplified by ever-prevalent ESBL-producing *K. pneumoniae* for which carbapenems were the mainstay treatment but are increasingly rendered ineffective by the sporadic emergence of carbapenem-resistant *Enterobacteriaceae* (CRE) [3,5,18].

Typical characteristics of ESBL-producing members of the *Enterobacteriaceae* family include resistance to amino- and carboxy-penicillins, second-generation cephalosporins and several third- and fourth-generation cephalosporins as well as monobactams (such as aztreonam) though some may remain susceptible to cephamycins [45,47,48,94,95]. Extended-spectrum β-lactamase producers additionally exhibit synergy between the former-mentioned antibiotics and clavulanate, a β-lactamase inhibitor, and may exhibit additional resistance towards other antibiotics, such as fluoroquinolones, aminoglycosides, trimethoprim and sulphamethoxazoles [2,11,14,47]. Treatment failure could be attributed to a drug's inability to reach therapeutic concentrations at the site of infection, particularly when the minimum inhibitory concentrations of the bacterium are close to the susceptibility breakpoint of drugs, such as ciprofloxacin sometimes used against temoneria (TEM)-52 ESBLs [91]. Empirical treatment should match information on pathogens distributed in the clinical setting and their respective susceptibility patterns so as to better ensure correct initial antimicrobial therapy [39]. Delayed appropriate treatment can increase the likelihood of death [39].

In a retrospective study conducted by Micek and colleagues (2010), a better outcome was believed to be associated with correct initial combination antimicrobial therapy when empirically treating Gram-negative bacteria-mediated sepsis as compared to monotherapy [92]. In the aforementioned study, a combination of a antipseudomonal fluoroquinolone, such as ciprofloxacin, or an aminoglycoside with a carbapenem (imipenem and meropenem), piperacillin-tazobactam or cefepime as initial treatment for severe Gram-negative bacterial infections offered a broader spectrum of activity [92]. Additional retrospective studies further favour combination therapy in CRE infections for which treatment options have been reduced mainly to colistin, tigecycline, some aminoglycosides and fosfomycin [4,18]. Although fosfomycin appears active *in vitro*, there is little clinical experience with the drug as well as knowledge of adequate combinations for treatment without encouraging antimicrobial resistance [4,96,97]. Tigecycline, on the other hand, has demonstrated effectiveness against MDR *Enterobacteriaceae* and despite requiring dosage adjustments, due to low blood levels, has good clinical experience [2,4,98]. An unfortunate drawback to tigecycline could include the selection of Gram-negative bacteria with efflux pump mutations [2,5]. Colistin has been recommended for use only in cases of known colistin-sensitive MDR strains or nosocomial and ICU late sepsis shock where MDR strains are suspected [4]. The use of colistin for a prolonged period (>13 days) of time has been suggested as responsible for the emergence of colistin-resistant or pandrug-resistant bacterial strains in some instances [17,99,100]. The emergence of MBL and KPC strains of *K. pneumoniae* has rendered them resistant to all but one antibiotic, namely colistin [101,102].

8. Antibiotic-resistance mechanisms in *K. pneumoniae* isolates

Innate antimicrobial susceptibility could be impacted by adaptive responses, resulting in alterations to gene expression and cell physiology, which are induced in response to the pathogen's natural environmental stresses or within a host [10,103–105] Three modes of antibiotic resistance existing in bacteria, such as *K. pneumoniae*, include drug modification or enzymatic inactivation, antibiotic target modification or decreased concentrations of antimicrobial drugs within cells (possible by reduced permeability) and increased efflux activity [9–11,106,107]. These modes of action are encoded either intrinsically or acquired through mutation and resistance gene acquisition [10,106]. The adaptive responses are not only triggered by antibiotics but can occur as a response to environmental stresses and include: (i) cessation of growth, (ii) stress-induced acquisition of resistance determinants, (iii) changes to target sites, (iv) altered membrane barrier functions, (v) induction of resistance-conferring mutations and (vi) promotion of biofilm formation [10,11,103]. Ironically, some protective responses activated as a result of the stress caused by antimicrobial drugs can lead to resistance towards these very same antimicrobial drugs [103,105].

Changes in membrane permeability and drug flux can be influenced by variable expression and regulation of the efflux pumps [11]. Within the *Enterobacteriaceae* Gram-negative bacteria, a significant bacterial efflux pump family is the resistance nodulation division (RND) [6,65,106,108]. The active expression of the chromosomal native AcrAB-TolC efflux pump of the RND family contributes to fluoroquinolone resistance in *E. coli*, *Enterobacter* spp. and *Klebsiella* spp [6,108,109]. Alternately, alterations in outer membrane proteins of both *K. pneumoniae* and *E. coli*, either due to mutations or deletion of porins, may limit influx of antimicrobial agents or alternately increase efflux [107]. Besides the major OmpK35 and OmpK36 porins, the alternative OmpK37, PhoE and LamB porins may be expressed by *K. pneumoniae* [110]. The latter three porins' role in antimicrobial resistance has not been thoroughly investigated but is suspected to be important in the absence of OmpK35 and OmpK36 [110]. Modification or loss of the OmpK35 and OmpK36 porin proteins can affect resistance in various ways either leading to elevated minimum inhibitory concentrations (MICs) or resistance towards carbapenems and expanded-spectrum cephalosporins, reduced fluoroquinolone susceptibility, or it may occasionally confer additional cross-resistance to quinolones, aminoglycosides and co-trimoxazole within broad-spectrum β-lactamase- or ESBL-producers [36,48,110–113]. An additional modification to the outer membrane aiding in resistance, other than porin loss, is the upregulation of capsule polysaccharide (CPS) production in *K. pneumoniae* [6,114].

Bacterial cells can exist as single cells, the planktonic form, or within communities drawn together by a self-produced biopolymer matrix and attached to a surface [46,105,115,116]. The latter is referred to as a biofilm and confers survival advantages in the form of improved resistance to host immune defences, resistance to biocides, increased resistance to antimicrobial compounds and higher plasmid transfer rates within that environment, which could include antibiotic resistance genes [10,46,75,115,116]. Genetic elements conferring potential resistance genes are easily transferred horizontally both intra- and interspecies due to the close genetic resemblance between bacteria of the *Enterobacteriaceae* family [10,11]. The reduced antimicrobial drug effect against bacterial populations within a biofilm is largely unclear but could be as a result of several mechanisms acting in conjunction, such as: (i) poor compound diffusion, (ii) the slower growth and uptake of antibiotics by the bacteria in mature biofilm (>24 hours old), (iii) the production of antimicrobial inactivating enzymes, (iv) general stress responses, (v) the expression of efflux pumps and (vi) the presence of persister cells (Figure 2.2) [10,46,105,115–117]. Biofilm formation in *K. pneumoniae* is influenced by cell density-dependent quorum sensing signalling *via* the non-specific bacterial type-2 QS regulatory molecules, AI-2 autoinducers [118]. The mannose-resistant *Klebsiella*-like (MR/K) haemagglutinins or "Mrk proteins" are encoded by the genes *mrk*ABCDF within an operon and form part of type 3 fimbriae, which is important in mediating biofilm formation in *K. pneumoniae* [119]. Antimicrobial drug resistance can increase up to 1000-fold for bacterial cells existing within the biofilm [115,120].

Finally, resistance towards β-lactam antibiotics are mainly mediated by β-lactamase enzyme production, which is capable of hydrolysing third-generation cephalosporins and monobactams [48,58,107,121,122]. Other factors at play besides ESBL production include cases of ESBL hyperproduction due to promoter upregulation after direct mutation, inserted transposable elements in close proximity to the promoter and the capacity of a strain to coproduce more than one ESBL [48].

9. Classification of β-lactamases

Enzyme-mediated resistance to β-lactam antibiotics was initially discovered in *E. coli* but has since spread to a large number of bacterial species in the form of over 890 unique β-lactamases [12]. Both the chromosomal and the plasmid encoded β-lactamases can be classified into either Bush-Jacoby-Medeiros functional groups based on hydrolysis and inhibition characteristics or four Ambler molecular classes based on the proteins' amino acid sequences, as illustrated in Table 1 [12,123]. The former Bush-Jacoby-Medeiros classifies the β-lactamases into three groups and 16 subgroups [6,12,123,124]. Some resistance genes exist through natural selection of resistant clonal lineages or have been acquired through mobile genetic elements, such as plasmids, transposons and insertion sequence elements (ISs) [23,24,125].

Functional group	Molecular class	Common name	Resistance to β-lactams
1	C	Cephalosporinase	Penicillins, cephalosporins, carbapenems*, monobactams*
2b	A	Penicillinase	Penicillins, early cephalosporins, β-lactamase inhibitor combinations*
2be	A	Extended-spectrum β-lactamase	Penicillins, cephalosporins, monobactams, β-lactamase inhibitor combinations
2d	D	Cloxacillinase	Penicillins (including oxacillin and cloxacillin)
2df	D	Carbapenemase	Carbapenems and other β-lactams
2f	A	Carbapenemase	All current β-lactams
3	B	Metallo-β-lactamase	All β-lactams, except monobactams

*β-lactams that are resistant as a function of high β-lactamase production in combination with efflux and porin modifications

Table 1. Major groups of β-lactamases in Gram-negative bacteria [12]

Ambler molecular classes A, C and D enzymes typically possess serine within the active site, while class B enzymes contain zinc [6,37,38,51]. Nine structural/evolutionary families have been described during the classification of ESBL variants [48]. The variants include Belgium extended-spectrum β-lactamase (BEL), Brazilian extended-spectrum β-lactamase (BES), CTX-M, Guyana extended-spectrum β-lactamase (GES), oxacillinase (OXA), *Pseudomonas* extended resistance (PER), *Serratia fonticola* (SFO), SHV, TEM, Tlahuicas (TLA) and Vietnam extended-spectrum β-lactamase (VEB) [6,14,48,126]. Other β-lactamases of importance are carbapenemases detected in *Enterobacteriaceae,* which typically include the OXA-48-type, KPC-type and MBL-type enzymes, Imipenem (IMP), Verona integron-encoded metallo-β-lactamases (VIM) and New Delhi metallo-β-lactamase (NDM) [20,37,127].

Three definitions of ESBLs have been proposed, which include a classical definition, a broadened definition and an all-inclusive definition [94]. The classical definition originally defined an ESBL as derivatives of broad-spectrum TEM and SHV enzymes and later more functionally defined as β-lactamases of the Ambler class A or functional group 2be capable of hydrolysing extended-spectrum cephalosporins and monobactams, while still being inhibited by β-lactamase inhibitors and poorly hydrolysing cephamycins and carbapenems [94]. The classical definition did not, on the other hand, account for the β-lactamases with similar hydrolysis profiles and dissimilar evolutionary backgrounds, such as CTX-M, GES and VEB enzymes [94]. A broader definition by Livermore (2008), included TEM and SHV variants with weaker ESBL activity, the enzymes with similar hydrolysis but dissimilar sources, as well as β-lactamases possessing wider resistance to the parent types that do not fall within the 2be functional group (e.g. OXA variants and AmpC type mutants). The wider resistance observed is to oxyimino-cephalosporins [94]. Lee and colleagues (2012) have independently extended the broadened definition of ESBLs to include AmpC ESBLs from the Ambler class C; thus designating ESBLs as: aESBLs, cESBLs and dESBLs [94]. The broadened definition is limited in that ESBLs with concurrent carbapenem and oxyimino-cephalosporin resistance are excluded [94].

Finally, the all-inclusive definition classifies ESBLs into three classes: $ESBL_A$ (class A ESBLs), $ESBLS_M$ (miscellaneous ESBLs including as AmpC and OXA-type ESBLs) and $ESBL_{CARBA}$ (β-lactamases encompassing ESBLs with carbapenem hydrolysing activity) [94,128]. The GES-1 β-lactamase, for example, has hydrolysis profiles resembling that of other ESBLs, but six GES β-lactamases have illustrated carbapenemase activity, being GES-2, -4, -5, -6, -11 and-14 [129]. Bush and colleagues (2009), on the other hand, felt the term $ESBL_{CARBA}$ as clinically confusing as ESBLs should be treatable with carbapenems and should thus remain more accurately classified as carbapenemases [130]. Bush and colleagues (2009) further disputes the definitions set by Giske (2009) by stating that AmpC-producers although treatable with carbapenems may develop resistance easily and should thus not be classified together with ESBLs [128,130]. The all-inclusive definition thus further excludes the clinical criteria in which ESBLs should have sensitivity to available β-lactamase inhibitors and current definitions of ESBLs, AmpC β-lactamases and carbapenemases should be kept independent [130]. The most common ESBL-encoding genes detected include SHV-, TEM- and CTX-M-type enzymes [6].

10. Risk factors for ESBL-producing *K. pneumoniae* infections

The clinical outcomes of inadequate empirical treatment with broad-spectrum antibiotics with no activity against the isolated causative bacterium (*in vitro*) or a bacterium with additional antibiotic resistance can lead to: (i) treatment failure, (ii) adverse patient outcomes, (iii) perpetuation of the increase in antimicrobial resistance and (iv) a financial burden to society [92,131]. The colonisation pattern in a patient after admission into hospital is largely influenced by the local antibiotic policy with increases in colonisation observed after 2 weeks, especially after treatment with broad-spectrum antibiotics, which lead to higher attack rates by nosocomial *K. pneumoniae* [59].

Generalised factors in at-risk patients commonly include severe illness, underlying medical conditions, recent surgery, haemodialysis, multiple or excessive antibiotic use, the use of medical devices, such as lines and tubes, prolonged hospitalisation, ICU admittance, admittance at long-term health facilities or nursing homes and international travel to endemic areas [132]. An important risk factor in modern society is the risk of acquiring ESBL-producing *K. pneumoniae* or *E. coli* when travelling to high-risk countries, particularly when travel is directed to endemic areas, such as to Asian countries or Greece, Turkey and the United States of America (USA), which have ESBLs and carbapenemases (such as KPC, VIM, OXA-48 and NDM) [45]. The risk of infection with ESBL-producing *E. coli* and *K. pneumoniae* is particularly higher if antibiotics were consumed during travel, often for traveller's diarrhoea [45,133].

The clinical manifestation of disease can be attributed to numerous host-dependent factors, which may range geographically but it is also influenced by socioeconomic determinants and the quality of healthcare at hand [26,27,89,90]. Underlying complications or illness that may result in an increased risk of *K. pneumoniae* infection include malignancy, cirrhosis, biliary tract disorders, diabetes mellitus and alcoholism [134].

11. Spread, prevention and control

The rise in antimicrobial-resistance among bacteria, such as those described as 'ESKAPE' pathogens (*Enterococcus faecium, Staphylococcus aureus, K. pneumoniae, A. baumannii, P. aeruginosa* and *Enterobacter* spp.), has highlighted the need for new antibiotics due to the 'escape' from currently marketed antimicrobial drugs [135]. The impact of infections with β-lactamase producing bacteria include increased mortality rates, particularly in blood stream infections (BSI), as well as increase in length of hospitalisation and hospital costs [2]. Principle reservoirs typically implicated in healthcare-associated outbreaks or spread includes the patients, the healthcare staff and the environment (such as sink drains) [21].

Factors impacting the spread and control of MDR bacteria include spread of plasmids and are impacted by the food chain or international travel [136]. During the travels, acquisition can occur in the absence of healthcare contact or along with leisure and medical tourism [45,137]. In healthcare settings, overcrowding is a key factor in exacerbating the faecal–oral route of transmission by either direct or indirect contact by healthcare workers [132]. The contact that staff have with patients during unassuming social interactions, such as taking a patient's blood pressure and the touching of inanimate objects in the patient's environment, could contribute to horizontal spread of pathogens, especially when elective hand hygiene practices are neglected [4,138]. The implementation of alcohol-based hand rubs and regular educational programmes are thus important steps in control measures undertaken [138]. The role of post-acute care facilities in dissemination of MDR bacteria is also stressed by Perez and colleagues (2010) [139].

Infection control measures undertaken can include: (i) increased barrier precautions, (ii) isolation of infected patients, (iii) appropriate antibiotic treatment duration and (iv) epidemiological standards for the handling of equipment as well as patient wounds [4,14,59]. A method investigated for its potential to reduce cross-contamination and infection rates in clinical settings, such as the ICU, is the effect of selective digestive tract decontamination (SDD) for the elimination of cephalosporin-resistant *Enterobacteriaceae* [140–143].

Several key shortcomings have, however, been identified by the World Health Organization (WHO) in the combat against antimicrobial resistance [144]. The issues are discussed under four topics which include: (i) lack of commitment and data, (ii) unconfirmed drug quality and irrational use, (iii) poor prevention and control of infections and (iv) languishing research into new antimicrobial agents and tools, including diagnostic tests and antimicrobials [144]. The resulting policy package recommended by the WHO thus firstly suggests that governments adopt and finance comprehensive national plans with accountability and engaging civil society by creating public awareness [144]. The second recommendation is based on improving surveillance and laboratory capacities, whilst the third advises local governments to guarantee an uninterrupted supply of essential, quality-assured medication [144]. The regulation and promotion of the correct use of former-mentioned medication is also emphasised along with good patient care [144]. Finally, the last two recommendations involve improvement of infection prevention and control while encouraging research and development of new tools, including diagnostic tests and antimicrobials [144].

12. Laboratory diagnosis of β-lactamase producing *K. pneumoniae* isolates

In light of increasing antibiotic resistance among bacteria, surveillance of drug-resistance patterns within clinical settings and clinically relevant pathogens is significant particularly when deciding on appropriate treatment for complicated infections [27]. The detection of ESBL-producing bacteria requires tests that can accurately discern between ESBL producers and bacteria possessing alternative resistance mechanisms, such as inhibitor-resistant-β-lactamases, cephalosporinase overproduction and SHV-1 hyperproduction [47].

12.1. Biochemical and phenotypic detection techniques

Characteristics associated with ESBL-producing *Enterobacteriaceae* include the synergy observable between the antibiotics amino- and carboxy-penicillins, second-generation cephalosporins and up to several third- and fourth-generation cephalosporins when combined with β-lactamase inhibitors, such as clavulanate [14,47]. *Klebsiella pneumoniae* can encode all three ESBL-encoding genes whilst simultaneously encoding carbapenemases [145]. The characteristics associated with KPC and MBL carbapenemase production differ to ESBLs in that the KPC enzyme is capable of hydrolysing all β-lactams, whereas the MBL enzymes are capable of hydrolysing all β-lactams but not aztreonam [127]. The former KPC β-lactamase is partially inhibited by inhibitors, such as boronic acid, clavulanic acid and tazobactam, whereas the latter MBL enzymes are inhibited by ethylene diamine tetra-acetate (EDTA) [127,146]. Detection of these MDR *K. pneumoniae* can be manually screened for utilising several techniques, which include culturing on chromogenic agar (such as ChromID® ESBL agar medium) (bioMérieux, France), Etest MBL (AB BioDisk Company, USA), MicroScan panels (MicroScan, USA), modified Hodge test, disk diffusion techniques on Mueller-Hinton agar and enriched medium (such as tryptic-soy broth containing 2 mg.L^{-1} cefpodoxime) [14,19,21,27,58,84]. Phenotypic techniques are often reliant on observable results, such as with the double disk synergy test (DDST), ESBL Etests (bioMérieux, France) and the combination disk method [47].

Initially, the DDST following methodology specified by the Clinical and Laboratory Standards Institute (CLSI) guidelines was intended for the differentiation between ESBL-producing *Enterobacteriaceae* strains and strains overproducing cephalosporinase, but the combination of cefotaxime or ceftazidime with clavulanic acid can also be predictive of a CTX-M-producer, particularly in *E. coli* [44,47]. The test makes use of a 30 μg disk of, e.g. cefotaxime and a disk of amoxicillin-clavulanate (10 μg clavulanate) approximately 30 mm apart, or at 20 mm for greater sensitivity [14,47]. The resistance breakpoints towards all third- and fourth-generation cephalosporins are not always apparent, regardless of whether disk diffusions in agar or automated systems are used [47]. False-negative results can occur when testing isolates encoding SHV-2, SHV-3 or TEM-12.[14] Alternatively, the ESBL Etests are capable of quantifying synergy with one end of the strip containing gradients of cefotaxime, or ceftazidime, or cefepime and the other end a combination of the same former-mentioned antibiotic with 4 $mg.L^{-1}$ clavulanate [47]. A limitation may include failure to detect ESBLs when ranges fall outside MIC ranges on the strip or misinterpretation of the inhibition ellipse [47,147,148]. Another phenotypic testing method that can be utilised is based on broth microdilution assays, which includes the commercially available MicroScan panels (Dade Behring MicroScan, Sacramento, USA) that make use of dehydrated panels for microdilution antibiotic susceptibility [14].

Cloxacillin has been added to agar media for the inactivation of cephalosporinases, an AmpC β-lactamase, whereas both clavulanate and EDTA have been added when MBLs are produced concurrently with ESBLs for the latter's identification and confirmation [47]. The detection of extended spectrum Ambler class D OXAs is, on the other hand, complicated due to weak inhibition and no inhibition observed towards clavulanate and EDTA, respectively [47,149]. A unique characteristic attributed to most class D β-lactamases, including OXA-48-type enzymes, is the inhibition of activity by sodium chloride (NaCl) *in vitro* at a concentration of 100 mM [49].

Carbapenemases can, on the other hand, also be screened for in at-risk patients using selective media, such as CHROMagar KPC medium (CHROMagar Ltd, France), Brilliance™ CRE medium (Thermo scientific, UK) and SUPERCARBA medium [127]. Typically, methods of detecting carbapenemases make use of inhibition tests utilising boronic acid, clavulanic acid, EDTA and tazobactam [112,127]. Carbapenemase resistance in *Enterobacteriaceae* can be confirmed phenotypically using the modified Hodge test (MHT) according to CLSI guidelines, although several limitations have been recorded [112]. Limitations include variable sensitivity and specificity recorded in the detection of carbapenemases other than KPC (>90% respectively) and the occurrence of false positive MHTs in the absence of carbapenemase production due to reduced susceptibility or resistance to carbapenems [112,150,151]. The latter limitation could be as a result of isolates expressing alternative mechanisms of carbapenem resistance, such as ESBL production coupled with loss of porin proteins [112,151]. The MHT test demonstrated good sensitivity in the detection of OXA-48-producers [152]. Inhibition-based carbapenemase detection is limited due to variable specificity and sensitivity [127].

12.2. Automated detection of ESBLs

Automated systems used for the detection of ESBLs are the VITEK®2 ESBL test (bioMérieux, France) and the Phoenix ESBL test (Becton Dickinson, USA), both of which monitor the bacterial growth response to expanded-spectrum cephalosporins [14,47]. The VITEK®2 ESBL test (bioMérieux, France) consists of cards with wells, whereas the automated Phoenix ESBL test (Becton Dickinson Biosciences, USA) consists of five wells containing a cephalosporin with or without clavulanic acid [47]. Another method that could be used for the detection of β-lactamase and carbapenemase activity is the matrix-assisted laser desorption ionization-time of flight (MALDI-TOF) mass spectrometry (MS), which analyse carbapenem molecule hydrolysis, although its efficiency in detecting OXA-48 producers remains uncertain [127,152–154].

12.3. Newer detection methods

Molecular investigations of outbreaks can be complicated when spurred by the spread of highly mobile plasmids [21]. Antimicrobial resistance genes are often carried on varied plasmids, which have been implicated in MDR Gram-negative bacteria outbreaks, as illustrated in a study by Tofteland and colleagues (2013), wherein the bla_{KPC} encoding plasmid was transmitted among varied strains and even species [21]. Non-phenotypic tests, including molecular techniques, that are available for antibiotic gene detection and typing include: polymerase chain reaction (PCR) assays, real-time PCR assays, next-generation sequencing (NGS) methodologies, microarrays, MALDI-TOF MS and PCR/electrospray ionization mass spectrometry (PCR/ESI MS) [127,152,155–158]. Molecular techniques, particularly PCR are the standard for detecting genes encoding ESBL, OXA-48-Like, VIM, KPC and NDM enzymes [50,152,159]. The detection of carbapenemases also includes the novel biochemical Carba NP test and a UV spectrophotometer-based technique [127,160,161]. The UV spectrophotometer-based method relies on the analysis of imipenem hydrolysis by extracted proteins from the isolate tested and demonstrates less variability in sensitivity (100%) and specificity (98.5%) as compared to inhibition-based methods [127,160,161]. Imipenem has also been used to detect carbapenemases using novel liquid chromatography-tandem mass spectrometry (LC-MS/MS) assays [162].

13. Typing of *K. pneumoniae* isolates

Genetic typing of *K. pneumoniae* isolates is important for outbreak investigations, investigating sources or reservoirs, understanding transmission, managing hospital infections and for epidemiological referencing [163–165]. Several typing methods exist for the characterisation of *K. pneumoniae* isolates, which can be subdivided into phenotypic and molecular methods, but the appropriate method used is dependent on the question that needs answering[28,29]. Originally, typing methods for *K. pneumoniae* included phenotypic typing methods, such as biotyping, serotyping, phage typing and bacteriocin typing [28,57,59,163,166,167]. The most popular serotyping method implemented in the past that gave the most reproducible results was capsule typing [59]. The technique was not, however, without its shortcomings as considerable serological cross-reactions could occur between the 77 capsule types [59]. Methods developed since then include molecular typing methods, such as amplified fragment length polymorphisms (AFLP), MALDI-TOF MS, MLST, multilocus variable-number tandem-repeat analysis (MLVA), NGS, pulsed field gel electrophoresis (PFGE), plasmid profiling, sodium dodecyl sulphate polyacryamide gel electrophoresis (SDS-PAGE), restriction fragment length polymorphism (RFLP), ribotyping and random PCR methods [28,29,57,62,163,165–168]. Random PCR methods include random amplified polymorphic DNA (RAPD) and repeat-based PCR (rep-PCR) [62].

The PFGE molecular method is highly discriminatory and is the gold standard typing method in the characterisation of *K. pneumoniae* isolates [163,164,169]. Pulsed-field gel electrophoresis discrimination is based on genomic DNA restriction utilising a rare-cutting restriction enzyme, such as *XbaI* for *K. pneumoniae* [29,170]. The disadvantage of PFGE lies in that intra-laboratory reproducibility of results requires substantial managing and it is technically demanding [164]. Multilocus sequence typing, on the other hand, is a useful technique utilised for determining the clonal relatedness between *K. pneumoniae* isolates and provides unambiguous, portable data [28,163,167]. The MLST and MLVA methods are both described numerically and much like MLST, the MLVA data are portable [29]. In MLST the internal segments of seven housekeeping genes in *K. pneumoniae* are amplified and the variations in each sequence described as unique alleles, which comprise the allelic profile of the isolate, otherwise known as a sequence type (ST) [29,167]. The disadvantage lies in that the discrimination may not be defining enough for outbreak analysis but it is useful to compare to global epidemiology [28, 29]. The MLVA, on the other hand, determines the number of repeat units at multiple loci and can be modified to the desired resolution depending on the loci chosen, thus allowing for a higher resolution than PFGE [29].

14. Commonly characterised *K. pneumoniae* strains

Sequence typing has allowed for the characterisation of *K. pneumoniae* strains and led to the recognition of widespread MDR clones [1,29]. Although a vast number of sequence types have been recorded globally, which can be accessed on public databases (such as www.pasteur.fr/mlst and http://pubmlst.org), a few important STs are frequently reported and discussed. Typing has elucidated widespread multidrug-resistant clones, such as *K. pneumoniae* ST 258, which can often produce KPC carbapenemases and the virulent *K. pneumoniae* clonal complex (CC) 23 (including ST 23 and ST 57) [21,23,29,30,171,172]. Besides the "classical" *K. pneumoniae* STs, a few STs associated with hvKP strains include ST 23 and ST 57, which are associated with the K1 capsular serotype, as well as the ST 86, ST 375 and ST 380, which are associated with the K2 capsular serotype [1,172]. It has been suggested that particular clones acquire resistance genes easily and may have evolutionarily changed similar genes acquired so as to maintain or improve bacterial fitness [173].

15. Conclusion

Enterobacteriaceae in the clinical setting have adapted to a harsh environment created by the use of antibiotics through several mechanisms, which include the expression of β-lactamases capable of hydrolysing penicillins as well as other β-lactam antimicrobials [6,12,54]. The β-lactamases commonly implicated in a range of serious infections by *K. pneumoniae* include cephalosporinases (particularly ESBLs) and carbapenemases [6]. Extended-spectrum-producing *K. pneumoniae* forms part of the ESBL-producing *Enterobacteriaceae*, which is collectively listed as one of six dangerous pathogens by the Infectious Disease Society of America together with *A. baumannii, P. aeruginosa,* vancomycin-resistant *E. faecium,* methicillin–resistant *S. aureus* and *Aspergillus* species. Other mechanisms of resistance and co-expression of several β-lactamases could work in concert to further extend the range of antimicrobial resistance by *K. pneumoniae,* often spurred on by excessive antimicrobial use in the clinical setting [10,11,103]. The consequences of the broadening resistance among Gram-negative bacilli, particularly towards the commonly implemented carbapenem antimicrobials, are often increased mortality rates and hospital costs, thus giving importance to tests with the capacity to discern between ESBLs, carbapenemases and other mechanisms of resistance being expressed [3,47,92]. The typing of bacterial isolates is also a paramount step in determining infection sources and possible dissemination routes [163,164,165].

Antibiotic resistance is often discussed in terms of selection and subsequent proliferation of MDR strains or the horizontal transfer of genetic elements encoding resistance, such as plasmids [30]. A combination of proteomics and molecular techniques could thus be used for the characterisation of plasmids within outbreak *K. pneumoniae* isolates [174]. Comparative studies of MDR bacterial proteomic information under specific *in vitro* conditions can also be used for the identification of proteins associated with antibiotic resistance [175]. Proteomic techniques could additionally be used for the investigation of possible immunogenic K. pneumoniae antigens, such as FepA (ferrienterobactin outer membrane receptor), OmpA (outer membrane protein A), OmpK36 (outer membrane porin) and the Colicin I receptor, for vaccine development [176,177]. Improving the understanding of the progression of drug resistance and mechanisms involved could aid attempts to improve the efficacy of current antimicrobials, an alternative solution in light of the lack of new drugs under development in recent years [3–5,175].

Author details

Marisa B. De Jesus[1], Marthie M. Ehlers[2], Ricardo F. Dos Santos[1] and Marleen M. Kock[2*]

*Address all correspondence to: marleen.kock@up.ac.za

1 Department of Medical Microbiology, University of Pretoria, Gauteng, South Africa

2 Department of Medical Microbiology, University of Pretoria and the National Health Laboratory Services (NHLS), Tshwane Academic Division, Gauteng, South Africa

References

[1] Shon AS, Bajwa RP, Russo TA. Hypervirulent (hypermucoviscous) Klebsiella pneumoniae a new and dangerous breed. Virulence 2013;4:1–12.

[2] Giske CG, Monnet DL, Cars O, Carmeli Y. Clinical and economic impact of common multidrug-resistant Gram-negative bacilli. Antimicrob Agent Chemother2008;52:813–21.

[3] Gasink LB, Edelstein PH, Lautenbach E, Synnestvest M, Fishman NO. Infection control and hospital epidemiology. Risk factors and clinical impact of Klebsiella pneumoniae carbapenemase-producing K. pneumoniae2009;30:1180–5.

[4] Giamarellou H. Multidrug-resistant Gram-negative bacteria: how to treat and for how long. Int J Antimicrob Agents2010;36:S50–4.

[5] Bush K. Improving known classes of antibiotics: an optimistic approach to the future. Curr Opin Pharmacol2012;12:527–34.

[6] Kocsis B, Szabó D. Antibiotic resistance mechanisms in Enterobacteriaceae. In: A Méndez-Vilas, ed. Microbial pathogens and strategies for combating them: science, technology and education. Spain: Formatex Research Center; 2013. pp. 251–257.

[7] Clegg S, Sebghati T. Klebsiella pneumoniae. In: Sussman M, edr. Molecular Medical Microbiology. California: Academic Press; 2001. pp. 1655–1680.

[8] Fertas-Aissani RE, Messai Y, Alouache S, Bakour R. Virulence profiles and antibiotic susceptibility patterns of Klebsiella pneumoniae strains isolated from different clinical specimens. Pathologie Biologie2013;61:209–16.

[9] Nordmann P, Poirel L. Acinetobacter baumannii – basic and emerging mechanisms of resistance. Eur Infect Dis2008;26:94–7.

[10] Fernández L, Breidenstein EBM, Hancock REW. Creeping baselines and adaptive resistance to antibiotics. Drug Resist Update2011;14:1–21.

[11] Kumar V, Sun P, Vamathevan J, Li Y, Ingraham K, Palmer L, Huang J, Brown JR. Comparative genomics of Klebsiella pneumoniae strains with different antibiotic resistance profiles. Antimicrob Agent Chemother2011;55:4267–76.

[12] Bush K. Bench to bedside review: the role of β-lactamases in antibiotic resistant Gram-negative infections. Critical Care2010;14:224–31.

[13] Khater ES, Sherif HW. Rapid detection of extended spectrum β-lactamase (ESBL) producing strain of Escherichia coli in urinary tract infections patients in Benha University Hospital, Egypt. Brit Microbiol Res J2014;4:443–53.

[14] Rawat D, Nair D. Extended-spectrum β-lactamases in Gram-negative bacteria. J Global Infect Dis2010;2:263–74.

[15] Gupta N, Limbago B, Patel J, Kallen AJ. Carbapenem-resistant Enterobacteriaceae: epidemiology and prevention. Clin Infect Dis2011;53:60–7.

[16] Brink A, Coetzee J, Clay C, Corcoran C, Van Greune J, Deetlefs JD, et al.. The spread of carbapenem-resistant Enterobacteriaceae in South Africa: risk factors for acquisition and prevention. S Afr Med J 2012;102:599–601.

[17] Brink AJ, Coetzee J, Corcoran C, Clay CG, Hari-Makkan D, Jacobson RK, et al. Emergence of OXA-44 and OXA-181 carbapenemases among Enterobacteriaceae in South Africa and evidence of in vivo selection of colistin resistance as a consequence of selective decontamination of the gastrointestinal tract. J Clin Microbiol2013;51:369–72.

[18] Van Duin D, Kaye KS, Neuner EA, Bonomo RA. Carbapenem-resistant Enterobacteriaceae: a review of treatment and outcomes. Diagnost Microbiol Infect Dis2013;75:115–20.

[19] Kitchel B, Rasheed JK, Patel JB, Srinivasan A, Navon-Venezia S, Carmeli Y, et al.. Molecular epidemiology of KPC-producing Klebsiella pneumoniae isolates in the United States: clonal expansion of multilocus sequence type 258. Antimicrob Agents Chemother2009;53:3365–70.

[20] Sisto A, D'Ancona F, Meledandri M. Pantosti A, Rossolini GM, Raglio A, et al. Carbapenem non-susceptible Klebsiella pneumoniae from Micronet network hospitals, Italy, 2009 to 2012 [Internet]. 2012. Available from: http://www.eurosurveillance.org/ViewArticle.aspx?ArticleId=20247 [Accessed: 6 October 2014]

[21] Tofteland S, Naseer U, Lislevand JH, Sundsfjord A, Samuelsen O. A long-term low-frequency hospital outbreak of KPC-producing K. pneumoniae involving intergenus plasmid diffusion and a persisting environmental reservoir. PLoS ONE2013;8:e59015.

[22] Storberg V. ESBL-producing Enterobacteriaceae in Africa - a non-systematic literature review of research published 2008-2012. Infect Ecol Epidemiol2014;4:10.3402/iee.v4.20342. DOI: DOI: 10.3402/iee.v4.20342

[23] Samuelsen Ø, Naseer U, Tofteland S, Skutlaberg DH, Onken A, Hjetland R, et al. Emergence of clonally related Klebsiella pneumoniae isolates of sequence type 258 producing plasmid-mediated KPC carbapenemase in Norway and Sweden. J Antimicrob Chemother2009;63:654–8.

[24] Grundmann H, Livermore DM, Giske CG, Canton R, Rossolini GM, Campos J, et al. Carbapenem-non-susceptible Enterobacteriaceae in Europe: conclusions from a meeting of national experts. Euro Surveill2010;15(46):pii:19711.

[25] Coetzee J, Brink A. The emergence of carbapenem resistance in Enterobacteriaceae in South Africa. S Afr J Epidemiol Infect2011;26:239–40.

[26] Yu VL, Hansen DS, Ko WC, Sagnimeni A, Klugman KP, Von Gottberg A, et al. Virulence characteristics of Klebsiella and clinical manifestations of Klebsiella pneumoniae bloodstream infections. Emerg Infect Dis2007;13:986–93.

[27] Bamford C, Bonorchis K, Ryan A, Simpson J, Elliott E, Hoffmann R, et al. Antimicrobial susceptibility patterns of selected bacteraemic isolates from South African public sector hospitals, 2010. S Afr J Epidemiol Infect2011;26:243–50.

[28] Diancourt L, Passet V, Verhoef J, Grimont PAD, Brisse S. Multilocus sequence typing of Klebsiella pneumoniae nosocomial isolates. J Clin Microbiol2005;43:4178–82.

[29] Woodford N, Turton JF, Livermore DM. Multiresistant Gram-negative bacteria: the role of high-risk clones in the dissemination of antibiotic resistance. FEMS Microbiol Rev2011;35:736–55.

[30] Chmelnitsky I, Shklyar M, Hermesh O, Navon-Venezia S, Edgar R, Carmeli Y. Unique genes identified in the epidemic extremely drug-resistant KPC-producing Klebsiella pneumoniae sequence type 258. J Antimicrob Chemother2013;68:74–83.

[31] Hoban DJ, Badal R, Bouchillon S, Hackel M, Kazmierczak K, Lascols C, et al. In vitro susceptibility and distribution of beta-lactamases in Enterobacteriaceae causing intra-abdominal infections in North America 2010-2011. Diagnost Microbiol Infect Dis2014;79:367–72.

[32] Gao L, Jiang X, Fu S, Gong H. In silico identification of potential virulence genes in 1,3-propanediol producer Klebsiella pneumoniae. J Biotechnol2014;189:9–14.

[33] Lery LMS, Frangeul L, Tomas A, Passet V, Almeida AS, Bialek-Davenet S, et al. Comparative analysis of Klebsiella pneumoniae genomes identifies a phospholipase D family protein as a novel virulence factor. BMC Biol2014;12:41.

[34] Yu WL, Chuang YC, Walther-Rasmussen J. Extended-spectrum beta-lactamases in Taiwan: epidemiology, detection, treatment and infection control. J Microbiol Immunol Infect2006;39:264–77.

[35] Derbyshire H, Kay G, Evans K, Vaughan C, Kavuri U, Winstanley T. A simple disc diffusion method for detecting AmpC and extended-spectrum β-lactamases in clinical isolates of Enterobacteriaceae. J Antimicrob Chemother2009;63:497–501.

[36] Ehlers MM, Veldsman C, Makgotlho EP, Dove MG, Hoosen AA, Kock MM. Detection of blaSHV, blaTEM, blaCTX-M antibiotic resistance genes in randomly selected bacterial pathogens from the Steve Biko Academic Hospital. FEMS Immonol Med Microbiol2009;56:191–6.

[37] Livermore DM. Defining an extended-spectrum β-lactamase. Clin Microbiol Infect2008;14:3–10.

[38] Falagas ME, Karageorgopoulos DE. Extended-spectrum β-lactamase-producing organisms. J Hospital Infect2009;73:345–54.

[39] Drugs and Therapeutics Bulletin (DTB). Risks of extended-spectrum beta-lactamases. Drugs Therapeut Bull2008;46:21–4.

[40] Livermore DM, Canton R, Gniadkowski M, Nordmann P, Rossolini GM, Arlet G, et al.CTX-M: Changing the face of ESBLs in Europe. J Antimicrob Chemother2007;59:165–74.

[41] Knothe H, Shah P, Krcmery V, Antal M, Mitshuhashi S. Transferable resistance to cefotaxime, cefoxitin, cefamandole and cefuroxime in clinical isolates of Klebsiella pneumoniae and Serratia marcescens. Infection1983;11:315–7.

[42] Sirot D, Sirot J, Labia R, Morand A, Courvalin P, Darfeuille-Michaud A, et al. Transferable resistance to third-generation cephalosporins in clinical isolates of Klebsiella pneumoniae: identification of CTX-1, a novel beta-lactamase. J Antimicrob Chemother1987;20:323–34.

[43] Philippon A, Labia R, Jacoby G. Extended-spectrum beta-lactamases. Antimicrob Agents Chemother1989;33:1131–6.

[44] Lewis JS, 2nd, Herrera M, Wickes B, Patterson JE, Jorgensen JH. First report of emergence of CTX-M-type extended-spectrum β-lactamases (ESBLs) as the predominant ESBL isolated in a U.S. health care system. Antimicrob Agents Chemother2007;51:4015–21.

[45] Van der Bij AK, Pitout JDD. The role of international travel in the worldwide spread of multiresistant Enterobacteriaceae. J Antimicrob Chemother2012;67:2090–100.

[46] Hennequin C, Aumeran C, Robin F, Traore O, Forestier C. Antibiotic resistance and plasmid transfer capacity in biofilm formed with a CTX-M-15-producing Klebsiella pneumoniae isolate. J Antimicrob Chemother2012;67:2123–30.

[47] Drieux L, Brossier F, Sougakoff W, Jarlier V. Phenotypic detection of extended-spectrum β-lactamase production in Enterobacteriaceae: review and bench guide. Clin Microbiol Infect2008;14:90–103.

[48] Gniadowski M. Evolution and epidemiology of extended-spectrum β-lactamases (ESBLs) and ESBL-producing microorganisms. Clin Microbiol Infect2001;7:597–608.

[49] Poirel L, Naas T, Nordmann P. Diversity, epidemiology and genetics of class D β-lactamases. Antimicrob Agents Chemother2010;54:24–38.

[50] Poirel L, Walsh TR, Cuvillier V, Nordmann P. Multiplex PCR for detection of acquired carbapenemase genes. Diagnost Microbiol Infect Dis2011;70:119–23.

[51] Hirsch E, Tam V.. Detection and treatment options for Klebsiella pneumoniae carbapenemases (KPCs): an emerging cause of multi-drug resistant infections. J Antimicrob Chemother2010;65:1119–25.

[52] National Institute for Communicable Diseases (NICD). Update on carbapenemase-producing Enterobacteriaceae. Communic Dis Communiq2013;12:5–6.

[53] Euzéby JP. List of Bacterial Names with Standing in Nomenclature: a folder available on the Internet. Int J Syst Bacteriol1997;47:590–2.

[54] Drancourt M, Bollet C, Carta A, Rousselier P. Phylogenetic analysis of Klebsiella species delineate Klebsiella and Raoultella gen. nov., with description of Raoultella ornithinolytica comb. nov., Raoultella terrigena comb. nov., and Raoultella planticola comb. nov.. Int J Syst Evolut Microbiol2001;51:925–32.

[55] UniProt: Taxonomy. Klebsiella pneumoniae [Internet]. 2014. Available from: http://www.uniprot.org/taxonomy/573 [Accessed: 3 October 2014]

[56] Leibniz Institut DSMZ-Deutsche Sammlung von Mikroorganismen und Zellkulturen GmbH: Bacterial Nomenclature Up-to-Date. Klebsiella [Internet]. 2012. Available from: http://www.dsmz.de/microorganisms/pnu/bacterial_nomenclature_info_mm.php?species=pneumoniae&bnu_no=777151&show_lit=1#777151 [Accessed: 24 October 2012]

[57] Brisse S, Verhoef J. Phylogenetic diversity of Klebsiella pneumoniae and Klebsiella oxytoca clinical isolates revealed by randomly amplified polymorphic DNA, gyrA and parC genes sequencing and automated ribotyping. Int J Syst Evolut Microbiol2001;51:915–24.

[58] Elhani D, Bakir L, Aouni M, Passet V, Arlet G, Brisse S, et al. Molecular epidemiology of extended-spectrum β-lactamase-producing Klebsiella pneumoniae strains in a university hospital in Tunis, Tunisia, 1999-2005. Clinic Microbiol Infect. 2010;16:157–64.

[59] Podschun R, Ullmann U. Klebsiella spp. as nosocomial pathogens: epidemiology, taxonomy, typing methods and pathogenicity factors. Clinic Microbiol Rev1998;11:589–603.

[60] Ørskov I. Genus V. Klebsiella Trevisan 1885, 105AL. In: Krieg NR, Holt JG, eds. Bergey's Manual of Systematic Bacteriology. Baltimore: Williams and Wilkins; 1984. pp. 461–5.

[61] Grimont PAD, Grimont F. Genus XVI Klebsiella. In: Brenner DJ, Krieg NR, Stanley JT, eds. Bergey's Manual of Systematic Bacteriology. New York: Springer; 2005. pp. 685–693.

[62] Brisse S, Grimont F, Grimont PAD. The Genus Klebsiella. Prokaryotes2006;6:159–96.

[63] Zhao L, Ma X, Zheng Y, Zhang J, Wei G, Wei D. Over-expression of glycerol dehydrogenase and 1,3-propanediol oxidoreductase in Klebsiella pneumoniae and their effects on conversion of glycerol into 1,3-propanediol in resting cell system. J Chem Technol Biotechnol2009;84:626–32.

[64] Marçal D, Rêgo AT, Carrondo MA, Enguita FJ. 1,3-Propanediol dehydrogenase from Klebsiella pneumoniae: decameric quaternary structure and possible subunit cooperativity. J Bacteriol2009;191:1143–51.

[65] Ramos P, Picão R, Almeida LG, Lima NC, Girardello R, Vivan AC, et al. Comparative analysis of the complete genome of KPC-2-producing Klebsiella pneumoniae Kp13

reveals remarkable genome plasticity and a wide repertoire of virulence and resistance mechanisms. BMC Genomics2014;15:54.

[66] Bai J, Liu Q, Yang Y, Wang J, Yang Y, Li J, et al. Insights into the evolution of gene organization and multidrug resistance from Klebsiella pneumoniae plasmid pKF3-140. Gene2013;519:60–6.

[67] Girlich D, Poirel L, Szczeponowski R, Schlüter A, Nordmann P. Carbapenem-hydrolyzing GES-5-encoding gene on different plasmid types recovered from a bacterial community in a sewage treatment plant. Appl Environment Microbiol2012;78:1292–5.

[68] Projan SJ. (Genome) Size matters. Antimicrob Agents Chemother2007;51:1133–4.

[69] Clements A, Gaboriaud F, Duval JFL, Farn JL, Jenney AW, Lithgow T, et al.. The major surface-associated saccharides of Klebsiella pneumoniae contribute to host cell association. PloS ONE2008;3:e3817.

[70] Johnson JG, Murphy CN, Sippy J, Johnson TJ, Clegg S. Type 3 fimbriae and biofilm formation are regulated by the transcriptional regulators MrkHI in Klebsiella pneumoniae. J Bacteriol2011;193:3453–60.

[71] Fuursted K, Scholer L, Hansen F, Dam K, Bojer MS, Hammerum AM, et al.. Virulence of a Klebsiella pneumoniae strain carrying the New Delhi metallo-β-lactamase-1 (NDM-1). Microbes Infect2012;14:155–8.

[72] Russo TA, Shon AS, Beanan JM, Olson R, MacDonald U, Pomakov AO, et al. Hypervirulent K. pneumoniae secretes more and more active iron-acquisition molecules than "classical" K. pneumoniae thereby enhancing its virulence. PloS ONE2011;6:e26734.

[73] Struve C, Bojer M, Krogfelt KA. Characterisation of Klebsiella pneumoniae type 1 fimbriae by detection of phase variation during colonization and infection and impact on virulence. Infect Immun2008;76:4055–65.

[74] Schembri MA, Blom J, Krogfelt KA, Klemm P. Capsule and fimbria interaction in Klebsiella pneumoniae. Infect Immunity2005;73:4626–33.

[75] Schroll C, Barken KB, Krogfelt KA, Struve C. Role of type 1 and type 3 fimbriae in Klebsiella pneumoniae biofilm formation. BMC Microbiol2010;10:179–88.

[76] Cortés G, Borrell N, De Astorza B, Gómez C, Sauleda J, Albertí S. Molecular analysis of the contribution of the capsular polysaccharide and the lipopolysaccharide O side chain to the virulence of Klebsiella pneumoniae in a murine model of pneumonia. Infection Immunity2002;70:2583–90.

[77] Moranta D, Regueiro V, March C, Llobet E, Margareto J, Garmendia J, et al. Klebsiella pneumoniae capsule polysaccharide impedes the expression of β-defensins by airway epithelial cells. Infection Immunity2010;78:1135–46.

[78] Pan YJ, Fang HC, Yang HC, Lin TL, Hsieh PF, Tsai FC, et al.. Capsular polysaccharide synthesis regions in Klebsiella pneumoniae serotype K57 and a new capsular serotype. J Clin Microbiol2008;46:2231–40.

[79] Turton JF, Baklan V, Siu LK, Kaufmann ME, Pitt TL. Evaluation of a multiplex PCR for detection of serotypes K1, K2 and K5 in Klebsiella sp. and comparison of isolates within these serotypes. FEMS Microbiol Lett2008;284:247–52.

[80] Brisse S, Fevre C, Passet V, Issenhuth-Jeanjean S, Tournebize R, Diancourt L, et al. Virulent clones of Klebsiella pneumoniae: identification and evolutionary scenario based on genomic and phenotypic characterization. Plos ONE2009;4:e4982.

[81] Pan YJ, Lin TL, Chen YH, Hsu CR, Hseih PF, Wu MC, et al. Capsular types of Klebsiella pneumoniae revisited by wzc sequencing. PLoS ONE2013;8:e80670.

[82] Yu WL, Ko WC, Cheng KC, Lee CC, Lai CC, Chuang YC. Comparison of prevalence of virulence factors for Klebsiella pneumoniae abscesses between isolates with capsular K1/K2 and non-K1/K2 serotypes. Diagnost Microbiol Infect Dis2008;62:1–6.

[83] Lascols C, Peirano G, Hackel M, Laupland KB, Pitout JDD. Surveillance and molecular epidemiology of Klebsiella pneumoniae isolates that produce carbapenemases: first report of OXA-48-Like enzyme in North America. Antimicrob Agents Chemother2013;57:130–6.

[84] Nordmann P, Poirel L, Carrër A, Tolemann MA, Walsh TR. How to detect NDM-1 producers. J Clin Microbiol2011;49:718–21.

[85] Lu CH, Chang WN, Chang HW. Klebsiella meningitis in adults: clinical features, prognostic factors and therapeutic outcomes. J Clin Neurosci2002;9:533–8.

[86] Wong CH, Kurup A, Wang YS, Heng KS, Tan KC. Four cases of necrotizing fasciitis caused by Klebsiella species. Eur J Clin Microbiol Infect Dis2004;23:403–7.

[87] Kohler JE, Hutchens MP, Sadow PM, Modi BP, Tavakkolizadeh A, Gates JD. Klebsiella pneumoniae and necrotizing fasciitis and septic arthritis: an appearance in the western hemisphere. Surgic Infection2007;8:227–32.

[88] Lin YT, Jeng YY, Chen TL, Fung CP. Bacteremic community-acquired pneumonia due to Klebsiella pneumoniae: clinical and microbiological characteristics in Taiwan, 2001-2008. BMC Infect Dis2010;10:307.

[89] Lautenbach E, Patel JB, Bilker WB, Edelstein PH, Fishman NO. Extended-spectrum β-lactamase–producing Escherichia coli and Klebsiella pneumoniae: risk factors for infection and impact of resistance on outcomes. Clin Infect Dis2001;32:1162–71.

[90] Ko WC, Paterson DL, Sagnimeni AJ, Hansen DS, Von Gottberg A, Mohapatra S, et al.. Community-acquired Klebsiella pneumoniae bacteremia: global differences in clinical patterns. Emerg Infect Dis2002;8:160–6.

[91] Endimiani A, Luzzaro F, Perilli M, Lombardi G, Coli A, Tamborini A, et al.. Bacteremia due to Klebsiella pneummoniae isolates producing TEM-52 extended-spectrum

β-lactamase: treatment outcome of patiemts receiving imipenem or ciprofloxacin. Clin Infect Dis2004;38:243–51.

[92] Micek ST, Welch EC, Khan J, Pervez M, Doherty JA, Reichley RM, et al.. Emperic combination antibiotic therapy is associated with improved outcome against sepsis due to Gram-negative bacteria: a retrospective analysis. Antimicrob Agents Chemother2010;54:1742–8.

[93] Vaara M. Polymyxins and their novel derivatives. Curr Opin Microbiol2010;13:574–81.

[94] Lee JH, Bae IK, Lee SH. New definitions of extended-spectrum β-lactamase conferring worldwide emerging antibiotic resistance. Med Res Rev2012;32:216–32.

[95] Breurec S, Guessennd N, Timinoni M, Le T, Cao V, Ngandjio A, et al.. Klebsiella pneumoniae resistant to third generation cephalosporins in five African and two Vietnamese major towns: multiclonal population structure with two major international clonal groups, CG15 and CG258. Clin Microbiol Infect2013;19:349–55.

[96] Falagas ME, Maraki S, Karageorgopoulos DE, Kastoris AC, Mavromanolakis E, Samonis G. Antimicrobial susceptibility of multidrug-resistant (MDR) and extensively drug resistant (XDR) Enterobacteriaceae isolates to fosfomycin. Int J Antimicrob Agents2010;35:240–3.

[97] Raz R. Fosfomycin: An old-new antibiotic. Clin Microbiol Infect2012;18:4–7.

[98] Souli M, Kontopidou FV, Koratzanis E, Antoniadou A, Giannitsioti E, Evangelopoulou P, et al. In vitro activity of tigecycline against multipledrug-resistant, including pan-resistant, Gram-negative and Gram-positive clinical isolates from Greek hospitals. Antimicrob Agents Chemother2006;50:3166–9.

[99] Antoniadou A, Kontopidou F, Poulakou G, Koratzanis E, Galani I, Papadomichelakis E, et al. Colistin-resistant isolates Klebsiella pneumoniae emerging in intensive care unit patients: first report of a multiclonal cluster. J Antimicrob Chemother2007;59:786–90.

[100] Mentzelopoulos SD, Pratikaki M, Platsouka E, Kraniotaki H, Zervakis D, Koutsoukou A, et al. Prolonged use of carbapenems and colistin predisposes to ventilator-associated pneumoniae by pandrug-resistant Pseudomonas aeruginosa. Intens Care Med2007;33:1524–32.

[101] Souli M, Kontopidou FV, Papadomichelakis E, Galani I, Armaganidis A, Giamarello H. Clinical experience of serious infections caused by Enterobacteriaceae producing VIM-1 metallo-beta-lactamases in a Greek university hospital. Clin Infect Dis2008;46:847–54.

[102] Souli M, Galani I, Antoniadou A, Papadomichelakis E, Poulakou G, Panagea T, et al. An outbreak of infection due to beta-lactamase Klebsiella pneumoniae carbapene-

mase 2-producing K. pneumoniae in a Greek university hospital: molecular characterisation, epidemiology and outcomes. Clin Infect Dis2010;50:364–73.

[103] Poole K. Bacterial stress responses as determinants of antimicrobial resistance. J Antimicrob Chemother2012;67:2069–89.

[104] Poole K. Stress responses as determinants of antimicrobial resistance in Gram-negative bacteria. Trend Microbiol2012;20:227–34.

[105] Bernier SP, Lebeaux D, DeFrancesco AS, Valomon A, Soubigou G, Coppée JY, et al. Starvation, together with the SOS response, mediates high biofilm-specific tolerance to the fluoroquinolone ofloxacin. PLoS Genet2013;9:e1003144.

[106] Poole K. Efflux-mediated multiresistance in Gram-negative bacteria. Clin Microbiol Infect2004;10:12–26.

[107] Page MGP, Dantier C, Desarbre E. In vitro properties of BAL30072, a novel siderophore sulfactam with activity against multiresistant gram-negative bacilli. Antimicrob Agents Chemother2010;54:2291–302.

[108] Poole K. Efflux-mediated antimicrobial resistance. J Antimicrob Chemother2005;56:20–51.

[109] Mazzariol A, Zuliani J, Cornaglia G, Rossolini GM, Fontana R. AcrAB efflux system: expression and contribution to fluoroquinolone resistance in Klebsiella spp. Antimicrob Agents Chemother2002;46:3984–6.

[110] García-Sureda L, Juan C, Doménech-Sánchez A, Albertí S. Role of Klebsiella pneumoniae LamB porin in antimicrobial resistance. Antimicrob Agents Chemother2011;55:1803–5.

[111] Wang XD, Cai JC, Zhou HW, Zhang R, Chen GX. Reduced susceptibility to carbapenems in Klebsiella pneumoniae clinical isolates associated with plasmid mediated β-lactamase production and OmpK36 porin deficiency. J Med Microbiol2009;58:1196–202.

[112] Carvalhaes CG, Picão RC, Nicoletti AG, Xavier DE, Gales AC. Cloverleaf test (modified Hodge test) for detecting carbapenemase production in Klebsiella pneumoniae: Be aware of false-positive results. J Antimicrob Chemother2010;65:249–51.

[113] Tsai YK, Fung CP, Lin JC, Chen JH, Chang FY, Chen TL, et al.. Klebsiella pneumoniae outer membrane porins OmpK35 and OmpK36 play roles in both antimicrobial resistance and virulence. Antimicrob Agents Chemother2011;55:1485–93.

[114] Campos MA, Vargas MA, Regueiro V, Llompart CM, Albertí S, Bengoechea JA. Capsule polysaccharide mediates bacterial resistance to antimicrobial peptides. Infect Immunity2004;72:7107–14.

[115] Mah TFC, O'Toole GA. Mechanisms of biofilm resistance to antimicrobial agents. Trends Microbiol2001;9:34–9.

[116] Soto SM. Role of efflux pumps in the antibiotic resistance of bacteria embedded in a biofilm. Virulence2013;4:223–9.

[117] Ito A, Taniuchi A, May T, Kawata K, Okabe S. Increased antibiotic resistance of Escherichia coli in mature biofilms. Appl Environ Microbiol2009;75:4093–100.

[118] De Araujo C, Balestrino D, Roth L, Charbonnel N, Forestier C. Quorum sensing affects biofilm formation through lipopolysaccharide synthesis in Klebsiella pneumoniae. Res Microbiol2010;161:595–603.

[119] Wilksch JJ, Yang J, Clements A, Gabbe JL, Short KR, Cao H, et al. MrkH, a novel c-di-GMP-dependent transcriptional activator, controls Klebsiella pneumoniae biofilm formation by regulating type 3 fimbriae expression. PLoS Pathogens2011;7:e1002204.

[120] De La Fuente-Núñez C, Reffuveille F, Fernández L, Hancock REW. Bacterial biofilm development as a multicellular adaptation: antibiotic resistance and new therapeutic strategies. Curr Opin Microbiol2013;16:580–9.

[121] Pitout JD, Hossain A, Hanson ND. Phenotypic and molecular detection of CTX-M-β-lactamases produced by Escherichia coli and Klebsiella spp. J Clin Microbiol2004;42:5715–21.

[122] Monstein H, Ostholm-Balkhed A, Nilsson MV, Nilsson M, Dornbusch K, Nilsson LE. Multiplex PCR amplification assay for the detection of blaSHV, blaTEM and blaCTX-M genes in Enterobacteriaceae. Acta Pathol, Microbiol Immunol Scandinav2007;115:1400–8.

[123] Ambler RP. The structure of β-lactamases. Philos Transac Royal Soc London Biol Sci1980;289:321–33.

[124] Bush K, Fisher JF. Epidemiological expansion, structural studies and clinical challenges of new β-lactamases from Gram-negative bacteria. Annu Rev Microbiol2011;65:455–78.

[125] Poirel L, Castanheira M, Carrër A, Rodriguez CP, Jones RN, Smayevsky J, et al.. OXA-163, an OXA-48-related class D β-lactamase with extended activity toward expanded-spectrum cephalosporins. Antimicrob Agents Chemother2011;55:2546–51.

[126] Naas T, Poirel L, Nordmann P. Minor extended-spectrum β-lactamases. Clin Microbiol Infect2008;14:42–52.

[127] Nordmann P, Poirel L. Strategies for the identification of carbapenemase-producing Enterobacteriaceae. J Antimicrob Chemother2013;68:487–9.

[128] Giske CG, Sundsfjord AS, Kahlmeter G, Woodford N, Nordmann P, Paterson DL, et al. Redefining extended-spectrum beta-lactamases: balancing science and clinical need. J Antimicrob Chemother2009;63:1–4.

[129] Patel G, Bonomo RA. “Stormy waters ahead”: global emergence of carbapenemases. Front Microbiol2013;4:48.

[130] Bush K, Jacoby GA, Amicosante G, Bonomo RA, Bradford P, Cornaglia G, et al. Comment on: redefining extended-spectrum beta-lactamases: balancing science and clinical need. J Antimicrob Chemother2009;64:212–5.

[131] Gudiol C, Tubau F, Calatayud L, Garcia-Vidal C, Cisnal M, Sánchez-Ortega I, et al.. Bacteraemia due to multi-drug resistant gram-negative bacilli in cancer patients: risk factors, antibiotic therapy and outcomes. J Antimicrob Chemother2011;66:657–63.

[132] Ghafourian S, Sadeghifard N, Soheili S, Sekawi Z. Extended spectrum beta-lactamases: definition, classification and epidemiology. Curr Issues Molecul Biol2014;17:11–22.

[133] Kuster SP, Hasse B, Huebner V, Bansal V, Zbinden R, Ruef C, et al. Risk factors for infection with extended-spectrum β-lactamase-producing Escherichia coli and Klebsiella pneumoniae at a tertiary care university hospital in Switzerland. Infection2010;38:33–40.

[134] Tsai SS, Huang JC, Chen ST, Sun JH, Wang CC, Lin SF, et al. Characteristics of Klebsiella pneumoniae bacteremia in community-acquired and nosocomial infections in diabetic patients. Chang Gung Med J2010;33:532–9.

[135] Boucher HW, Talbot GH, Bradley JS, Edwards JE, Gilbert D, Rice LB, et al. Bad bugs, no drugs: no ESKAPE! An update from the Infectious Diseases Society of America. Clin Infect Dis2009;48:1–12.

[136] Kluytmans-van den Bergh MF, Kluytmans JA. Editorial commentary: control of multidrug-resistant microorganisms: beyond the hospital. Clin Infect Dis2012;55:1512–4.

[137] Rogers BA, Aminzadeh Z, Hayashi Y, Paterson DL. Country-to-country transfer of patients and the risk of multi-resistant bacterial infection. Clin Infect Dis2011;53:49–56.

[138] Allegranzi B, Pittet D. Role of hand hygiene in healthcare-associated infection prevention. J Hospital Infect2009;73:305–15.

[139] Perez F, Endimiani A, Ray AJ, Decker BK, Wallace CJ, Hujer KM, et al. Carbapenem-resistant Acinetobacter baumannii and Klebsiella pneumoniae across a hospital system: impact of post-acute care facilities on dissemination. J Antimicrob Chemother2010;65:1807–18.

[140] De Smet AM, Kluytmans JA, Cooper BS, Mascini EM, Benus RF, Van der Werf TS, et al. Decontamination of the digestive tract and oropharynx in ICU patients. New Engl J Med2009;360:20–31.

[141] De Smet AM, Kluytmans JA, Blok HE, Mascini EM, Benus RF, Bernards AT, et al. Selective digestive tract decontamination and selective oropharyngeal decontamination and antibiotic resistance in patients in intensive-care units: an open-label, clusters group-randomised, crossover study. Lancet Infect Dis2011;11:372–80.

[142] Oostdijk EA, De Smet AM, Kesecioglu J, Bonten MJ, Dutch SOD-SDD Trialist Group. The role of intestinal colonisation with Gram-negative bacteria as a source for intensive care unit-acquired bacteremia. Crit Care Med2011;39:961–6.

[143] Oostdijk EA, De Smet AM, Kesecioglu J, Bonten MJ. Decontamination of cephalosporin-resistant Enterobacteriaceae during selective digestive tract decontamination in intensive care units. J Antimicrob Chemother2012;67:2250–3.

[144] Leung E, Weil DE, Raviglione M, Nakatani H, World Health Organisation World Health Day Antimicrobial Resistance Technical Working Group. The WHO policy package to combat antimicrobial resistance. Bull World Health Organizat2011;89:390–2.

[145] Cabral AB, Melo R, Maciel MA, Lopes AC. Multidrug resistance genes, including blaKPC and blaCTX-M-2, among Klebsiella pneumoniae isolated in Recife, Brazil. Revist Socie Brasil Med Tropical2012;45:572–8.

[146] Nordmann P, Gniadkowski M, Giske CG, Poirel L, Woodford N, Miriagou V, et al.. Identification and screening of carbapenemase-producing Enterobacteriaceae. Clin Microbiol Infect2012;18:432–8.

[147] Carter MW, Oakton KJ, Warner M, Livermore DM. Detection of extended-spectrum beta-lactamases in klebsiellae with the Oxoid combination disk method. J Clin Microbiol2000;38:4228–32.

[148] Leverstein-van Hall MA, Fluit AC, Paauw A, Box AT, Brisse S, Verhoef J. Evaluation of the Etest ESBL and the BD Phoenix, VITEK 1 and VITEK 2 automated instruments for the detection of extended-spectrum beta-lactamases in multiresistant Escherichia coli and Klebsiella spp. J Clin Microbiol2002;40:3703–11.

[149] Naas T, Nordmann P. OXA-type beta-lactamases. Curr Pharmaceut Design1999;5:865–79.

[150] Centers for Disease Control and Prevention (CDC). Laboratory protocol for detection of carbapenem-resistant or carbapenemase-producing Klebsiella spp. and E. coli from rectal swabs [Internet]. 2008. Available from: http://www.cdc.gov/HAI/settings/lab/lab_settings.html or http://www.cdc.gov/HAI/pdfs/labSettings/Klebsiella_or_Ecoli.pdf [Accessed: 11 June 2014]

[151] Clinical and Laboratory Standards Institute. Performance standards for antimicrobial susceptibility testing: Twenty-fourth informational supplement M100-S24. Wayne, PA, USA: CLSI; 2014.

[152] Poirel L, Potron A, Nordmann P. OXA-48-Like carbapenemases: the phantom menace. J Antimicrob Chemother2012;67:1597–606.

[153] Burckhardt I, Zimmermann S. Using matrix–assisted laser desorption ionisation-time of flight mass spectrometry to detectcarbapenem resistance within 1 to 2.5 hours. J Clin Mircobiol2011;49:3321–4.

[154] Hrabák J, Chudácková E, Walková R. Matrix-assisted laser desorptionionisation-time of flight (MALDI-TOF) mass spectrometryfor detection of antibiotic resistance mechanisms: from research to routine diagnosis. Clin Microbiol Rev2013;26:103–14.

[155] Dallenne C, Da Costa A, Decré D, Favier C, Arlet G. Development of a set of multiplex assays for detection of genes encoding important β-lactamases in Enterobacteriaceae. J Antimicrob Chemother2010;65:490–5.

[156] Voets GM, Fluit AC, Scharringa J, Stuart JC, Leverstein-van Hall MA. A set of multiplex PCRs for the genotypic detection of extended-spectrum β-lactamases, carbapenemases, plasmid-mediated AmpC β-lactamases and OXA β-lactamases. Int J Antimicrob Agents2011;37:356–9.

[157] Lupo A, Papp-Wallace KM, Sendi P, Bonomo RA, Endimiani A. Non-phenotypic tests to detect and characterize antibiotic resistance mechanisms in Enterobacteriaceae. Diagnost Microbiol Infect Dis 2013;77:179–94.

[158] Veenemans J, Overdevest IT, Snelders E, Willemsen I, Hendriks Y, Adesokan A, et al. Next-generation sequencing for typing and detection of resistance genes: performance of a new commercial method during an outbreak of extended-spectrum-beta-lactamase-producing Escherichia coli. J Clin Microbiol2014;52:2454–60.

[159] Avlami A, Bekris S, Ganteris G, Kraniotaki E, Malamou-Lada E, Orfanidou M, et al. Detection of metallo-β-lactamase genes in clinical specimens by a commercial multiplex PCR system. J Microbiol Methods2010;83:185–7.

[160] Bernabeu S, Poirel L, Nordmann P. Spectrophotometry-based detection of carbapenemase producers in Enterobacteriaceae. Diagnost Microbiol Infect Dis2012;74:88–90.

[161] Nordmann O, Poirel L, Dortel L. Rapid detection of carbapenemase producing Enterobacteriaceae. Emerg Infect Dis2012;18:1503–7.

[162] Kulkarni MV, Zurita AN, Pyka JS, Murray TS, Hodsdon ME, Peaper DR. Use of imipenem to detect KPC, NDM, OXA, IMP and VIM carbapenemase activity from Gram-negative rods in 75 minutes using liquid chromatography-tandem mass spectrometry. J Clin Microbiol2014;52:2500–5.

[163] Johnson JK, Arduino SM, Stine OC, Johnson JA, Harris AD. Multilocus sequence typing compared to pulsed-field gel electrophoresis for molecular typing of Pseudomonas aeruginosa. J Clin Microbiol2007;45:3707–12.

[164] Vimont S, Mnif B, Fevre C, Brisse S. Comparison of PFGE and multilocus sequence typing for analysis of Klebsiella pneumoniae isolates. J Med Microbiol2008;57:1308–10.

[165] Berrazeg M, Diene SM, Drissi M, Kempf M, Richet H, Landraud L, et al. Biotyping of multidrug-resistant Klebsiella pneumoniae clinical isolates from France and Algeria using MALDI-TOF MS. PLoS ONE.2013;8:e61428.

[166] Brisse S, Issenhuth-Jeanjean S, Grimont PA. Molecular serotyping of Klebsiella species isolates by restriction of the amplified capsular antigen gene cluster. J Clin Microbiol2004;42:3388–98.

[167] Aanensen DM, Spratt BG. The multilocus sequence typing network: mlst.net. Nucleic Acids Res2005;33:W728–33.

[168] Arena F, Rolfe PA, Doran G, Conte V, Gruszka S, Clarke T, et al. Rapid resistome fingerprinting and clonal lineage profiling of carbapenem-resistant Klebsiella pneumoniae isolates by targeted next-generation sequencing. J Clin Microbiol2014;52:987–90.

[169] Hansen DS, Skov R, Benedi JV, Sperling V, Kolmos HJ. Klebsiella typing: pulsed-field gel electrophoresis (PFGE) in comparison with O:K-serotyping. Clin Microbiol Infect2002;8:397–404.

[170] Durmaz R, Otlu B, Koksal F, Hosoglu S, Ozturk R, Ersoy Y, et al. The optimization of a rapid pulsed-field gel electrophoresis protocol for typing of Acinetobacter baumannii, Escherichia coli and Klebsiella spp. Jpn J Infect Dis2009;62:372–7.

[171] Baraniak A, Izdebski R, Herda M, Fiett J, Hryniewicz W, Gniadkowski M, et al. Emergence of Klebsiella pneumoniae ST258 with KPC-2 in Poland. Antimicrob Agents Chemother2009;53:4565–7.

[172] Merlet A, Cazanave C, Dutronc H, Barbeyrac B, Brisse S, Dupon M. Primary liver abscess due to CC23-K1 virulent clone of Klebsiella pneumoniae in France. Clin Microbiol Infect2012;18:E338–9.

[173] Deschamps C, Clermont O, Hipeaux MC, Arlet G, Denamur E, Branger C. Multiple acquisitions of CTX-M plasmids in the rare D2 genotype of Escherichia coli provide evidence for convergent evolution. Microbiology2009;155:1656–68.

[174] Lau AF, Wang H, Weingarten RA, Drake SK, Suffredini AF, Garfield MK, et al. A rapid matrix–assisted laser desorption ionisation-time of flight mass spectrometry-based methods for single–plasmid tracking in an outbreak of carbapenem-resistant Enterobacteriaceae. J Clin Microbiol2014;52:2804–12.

[175] Vranakis I, Goniotakis I, Psaroulaki A, Sandalakis V, Tselentis Y, Gevaert K, et al. Proteome studies of bacterial antibiotic resistance mechanisms. J Proteomics2014;97:88–99.

[176] Kurupati P, Teh BK, Kumarasinghe G, Poh CL. Identification of vaccine candidate antigens of an ESBL producing Klebsiella pneumoniae clinical strain by immunoproteome analysis. Proteomics2006;6:836–44.

[177] Lundberg U, Senn BM, Schüler W, Meinke A, Hanner M.. Identification and characterisation of antigens as vaccine candidates against Klebsiella pneumoniae. Human Vaccines Immunother2013;9:497–505.

Chapter 5

Antimicrobial Resistance in Staphylococci at the Human–Animal Interface

Tracy Schmidt, Marleen M. Kock and Marthie M. Ehlers

Additional information is available at the end of the chapter

http://dx.doi.org/10.5772/61785

Abstract

The widespread and often indiscriminate use of antimicrobials in animals is considered an important driving force behind the emergence and spread of antimicrobial-resistant bacteria. The emergence of livestock-associated methicillin-resistant *Staphylococcus aureus* and the description of a novel methicillin-resistant gene, *mec*C, have renewed concerns regarding the role of animals as reservoirs and a source for the evolution of novel, virulent zoonotic pathogens. The transfer of antimicrobial-resistant bacteria residing in, or on, animals to close human contacts or the introduction of the bacteria into the food supply chain is a cause for concern. The purpose of this mini-review is to provide a background to the genus *Staphylococcus* and the emergence of antimicrobial resistance as well as a discussion on the most significant antimicrobial resistance mechanisms. The use of antimicrobials in animal husbandry is discussed and the interface between humans and different animal populations is closely examined. Finally, the need for antimicrobial monitoring programmes is discussed and is supplemented with information pertaining to antimicrobial susceptibility testing and molecular typing of staphylococcal isolates.

Keywords: Staphylococci, Antimicrobial Resistance, MRSA, LA-MRSA, Animals

1. Introduction

Staphylococci are natural residents on the skin and mucous membranes of a wide range of host species [1]. Many of the bacterial species have a benign or symbiotic relationship with their host; however, the bacteria may become pathogenic if they gain entry into the host tissue through trauma of the cutaneous barrier [2, 3]. *Staphylococcus aureus* is the most significant species within this genus by virtue of its versatility as a pathogen in humans and animals [4, 5]. In humans, *S. aureus* is responsible for a variety of conditions, ranging from superficial skin infections to life-threatening diseases [6]. In addition, through the production of potent

INTECH
open science | open minds

© 2015 The Author(s). Licensee InTech. This chapter is distributed under the terms of the Creative Commons Attribution License (http://creativecommons.org/licenses/by/3.0), which permits unrestricted use, distribution, and reproduction in any medium, provided the original work is properly cited.

superantigens and other toxins, *S. aureus* can cause specific toxin-mediated conditions such as toxic shock syndrome, scalded skin syndrome and food poisoning [6]. In animals, *S. aureus* is a common cause of intramammary infections (IMIs), or mastitis [7]. Worldwide, the dairy industry incurs significant financial losses annually due to intramammary infections [8–10].

Other *Staphylococcus* species, collectively termed coagulase-negative staphylococci (CNS), are responsible for a variety of opportunistic infections in humans and animals [11]. Due to the ubiquity of many of the species within this group, their clinical significance has traditionally been dismissed, and when isolated from clinical specimens, the bacteria have merely been regarded as contaminants [12]. This perception is, however, changing as many species have emerged as important causes of nosocomial infections, particularly in relation to foreign-device-related infections and infections in immunocompromised patients [1, 13].

The propensity for staphylococci to develop antimicrobial resistance is a cause for great concern in both human and veterinary medicine [14]. As the efficacy of antimicrobials declines, the morbidity and mortality in infected patients increase [15, 16]. Moreover, in the case of human medicine, the costs associated with the treatment of infections caused by antimicrobial-resistant bacteria represent a serious public health burden in hospital and community settings [10].

2. The genus *Staphylococcus*

2.1. Classification of staphylococci

Before the 1970s, *S. aureus* and *S. epidermidis*, or *S. albus* as it was originally named, were the only recognized *Staphylococcus* species [17]. *Staphylococcus aureus* was considered a pathogen and *S. epidermidis*, when isolated from clinical material, was regarded as a contaminant [17]. In the mid-1970s, Kloos and Schleifer [17–19] conducted comprehensive systematic studies of staphylococci and micrococci and described a number of new species. To date, 49 species and 26 subspecies have been described and with improvements in the accuracy of genotyping methods the number of species is still increasing [20, 21].

The genus *Staphylococcus* is classified along with the genera *Jeotgalicoccus, Macrococcus, Nosocomiicoccus* and *Salinicoccus* in the family *Staphylococcaceae* [12, 21]. The full Linnaean classification for the genus and the type species, *S. aureus*, is shown in Table 1.

In diagnostic laboratories, staphylococci are historically differentiated by their ability to produce the enzyme coagulase, which mediates the conversion of fibrinogen to fibrin resulting in the clotting of blood [22]. The production of coagulase has long been recognized as an important indicator of pathogenicity [23, 24], and the coagulation of rabbit plasma provides a rapid *in vitro* method for differentiating pathogenic coagulase-positive staphylococci (CPS) and 'non-pathogenic' coagulase-negative staphylococci [1, 24].

Seven CPS are currently recognized, namely *S. aureus, S. lutrae, S. schleiferi* subsp. *coagulans*, the coagulase-variable, *S. hyicus* and the *S. intermedius* group (SIG), which comprises *S.*

Taxonomy	Name
Domain	*Bacteria*
Kingdom	*Eubacteria*
Phylum	*Firmicutes*
Class	*Bacilli*
Order	*Bacillales*
Family	*Staphylococcaceae*
Genus	*Jeotgalicococcus* *Macrococcus* *Nosocomiicoccus* *Salinococcus* *Staphylococcus*
Species	*Staphylococcus aureus*
Subspecies	*Staphylococcus aureus* subsp. *aureus* *Staphylococcus aureus* subsp. *anaerobius*

Table 1. The current Linnaean classification scheme for the genus *Staphylococcus* [21].

intermedius, *S. pseudintermedius* and *S. delphini* [25, 26]. *Staphylococcus aureus*, which is known to be pathogenic in both humans and animals, is considered to be the most important of all the CPS. Other CPS, particularly *S. hyicus* and members of the SIG group, are important veterinary pathogens and are responsible for infections in a number of different animal species [2, 25, 26].

The CNS comprise a biochemically heterogeneous group of bacteria which have, for convenience, been grouped together by virtue of their inability to produce the enzyme coagulase [23, 24]. The susceptibility of CNS isolates to novobiocin has been shown to be a useful phenotypic characteristic in diagnostic laboratories to differentiate *S. saprophyticus* from other clinically important species [2, 27]. The phylogenetic relationship between the coagulase-negative staphylococcal species has recently been clarified through the analysis of four gene loci, namely the 16S rRNA gene and the three protein-encoding genes, *dnaJ*, *rpoB* and *tuf*, which code for heat shock protein 40, the β-subunit of RNA polymerase and elongation factor Tu, respectively [12, 28]. The molecular analysis resolved the CNS into 14 cluster groups, which are depicted in Figure 1.

2.2. General characteristics of staphylococci

Staphylococci are non-motile, non-sporeforming Gram-positive coccus-shaped bacteria [29]. The cocci may occur singly, in pairs and in tetrads, and they characteristically divide in more than one plane to form irregular 'grape-like' clusters [2, 29]. In fact, the name *Staphylococcus* is derived from the Greek words '*staphyle*' and '*kokkos*' meaning 'bunch of grapes' and 'berry', respectively [1, 29]. Most staphylococci are facultative anaerobes and catalase positive with

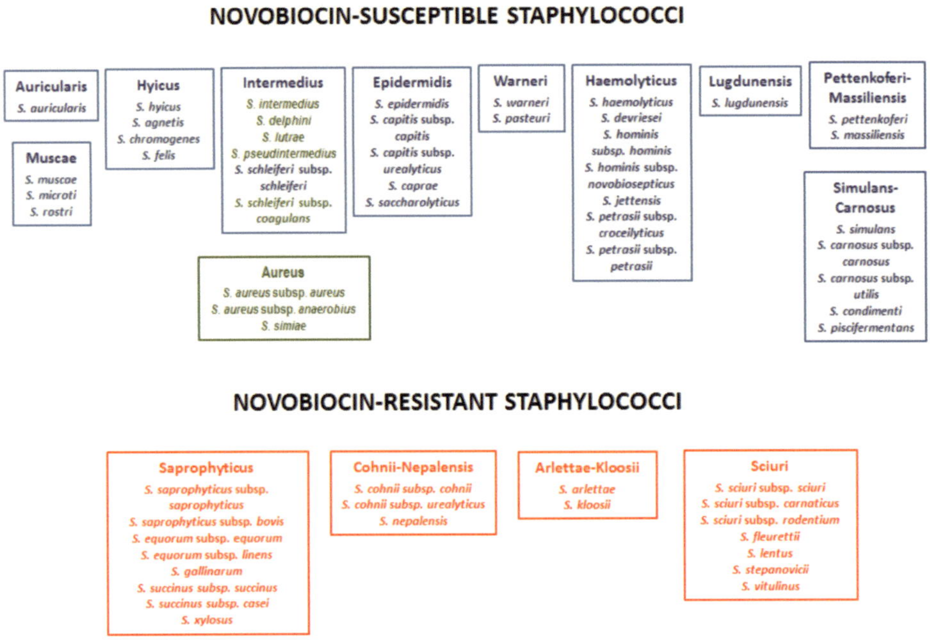

Figure 1. Phylogenetic separation of staphylococcal species and subspecies. Coagulase-positive *Staphylococcus* spp. are shown in green font [12, 28].

the exception of *S. aureus* subsp. *anaerobius* and *S. saccharolyticus* [1]. Staphylococci can grow in a wide pH range (4.8–9.4) and can survive temperatures of up to 60°C for 30 minutes [29]. Many *Staphylococcus* species are tolerant of high salt concentrations (7.5–10%) due to the production of osmoprotectants [29]. The ability to grow in the presence of above-average salt concentrations explains the predilection of many staphylococcal species for the sebaceous surfaces of mammals [1]. This phenotypic trait is exploited in diagnostic laboratories by incorporating high concentrations of sodium chloride into agar media to selectively isolate staphylococci from contaminated samples [1, 5].

Staphylococcus aureus is able to exist as a commensal on the skin and mucous membranes of different hosts, but when the opportunity presents, the bacterium is able to become pathogenic [1]. *Staphylococcus aureus* can colonize a number of sites on the human body with the anterior nares being the preferred site [30, 31]. Approximately 20% of healthy humans are persistent nasal carriers of *S. aureus*, about 30% are intermittent carriers and around 50% of individuals are never colonized with *S. aureus* [31, 32]. Individuals who are colonized by *S. aureus* are at a higher risk of becoming infected and are also an important source for the dissemination of *S. aureus* among individuals in the community [1, 33]. The primary means of transmission of *S. aureus* is by direct contact, usually skin-to-skin contact with colonized or infected individuals, although indirect means, via fomites, is also thought to play a role [33]. Various host factors, including loss of the normal skin barrier, the presence of underlying diseases, such as diabetes and acquired immunodeficiency syndrome, predispose individuals to infection [33].

The success of *S. aureus* as a pathogen is attributed in part to the capacity of the bacteria to produce a diverse array of virulence factors [1, 14]. Some of these factors may be more important than others in different diseases or at different stages of pathogenesis as not all factors are produced by each strain [34, 35]. Based on structure and functionality, the virulence factors can be broadly divided into two general groups, namely surface-associated factors and degradative enzymes, including exotoxins [36]. The microbial surface components of *S. aureus* recognizing the adhesive matrix molecular components (MSCRAMMs) comprise surface proteins that promote colonization by binding to host cells [36]. This group, which includes fibrinogen-, fibronetin- and collagen-binding proteins, is important during the initial stage of infection [37]. Once infection is established, the expression of tissue-binding proteins is downregulated, whilst the synthesis of extracellular toxins and tissue-degrading enzymes is induced to aid the acquisition of nutrients and the dissemination of the bacteria [38].

The CNS constitute a significant proportion of the natural microflora colonizing the skin and mucous membranes of humans and animals [12, 39]. The different staphylococcal species display apparent site or niche preferences on their hosts and occur more frequently at these sites [2, 12]. *Staphylococcus epidermidis* is the most abundant and widely distributed species on human skin and can occur in densities of 10^3 to 10^4 cells cm^{-2} [12, 40, 41]. *Staphylococcus epidermidis* is particularly prevalent in moist areas, such as the axillae, inguinal and perineal areas, anterior nares, conjunctiva and toe webs [12]. *Staphylococcus haemolyticus* and *S. hominis* are preferentially isolated from areas of the skin where there are numerous apocrine glands such as the axillae and pubic areas, whereas *S. capitis* is typically located around the sebaceous glands on the forehead and scalp following puberty [2, 12]. *Staphylococcus warneri* is commonly recovered from human hands, whilst *S. lugdunensis* has a preference for the inguinal and breast areas [41–43].

Coagulase-negative staphylococci are typically less pathogenic than *S. aureus* possessing a smaller array of virulence factors [12]. However, CNS often exhibit greater resistance to antimicrobials and also have a greater tendency to develop multidrug resistance [44]. Coagulase-negative staphylococci are believed to serve as reservoirs of antimicrobial resistance genes, which can transfer and integrate into the *S. aureus* genome leading to the emergence of new, potentially more resistant strains [45, 46].

3. Genomic organization and genetic flexibility of *S. aureus*

The staphylococcal genome consists of a closed circular molecule of double-stranded DNA between two and three megabase pairs in length and encoding between 2 509 and 2 892 open-read frames [1, 47]. Whole genome sequencing of a number of *S. aureus* strains has revealed that approximately 75% of the bacterium's genome comprises a core component, common to all strains [6]. The majority of the genes comprising the core genome are those associated with central metabolism and other housekeeping functions [48]. The remaining 25% of the *S. aureus* genome, termed the accessory genome, contains genes that encode a diverse array of non-essential functions ranging from virulence, antimicrobial and metal resistance, to substrate utilization and miscellaneous metabolism [49]. Many of the regions making up the accessory genome are, or once were, mobile genetic elements (MGEs), such as chromosomal cassettes, pathogenicity islands, plasmids, prophages and transposons [50]. Mobile genetic elements can be transferred horizontally between bacteria of the same or different species, leading to the evolution of bacterial strains [50, 51]. The distribution of these elements is therefore important from a clinical perspective, as it may lead to the evolution of bacterial strains that are potentially more virulent or resistant to antimicrobials [50].

3.1. Host specificity and host switching of *S. aureus*

Devriese and Oeding [52] were amongst the first researchers to note the occurrence of phenotypic differences between *S. aureus* strains isolated from humans and different animal hosts. A simplified biotyping scheme was developed by Devriese and co-workers to differentiate *S. aureus* isolates into ecological variants, or ecovars, that delineated along human, poultry or ruminant associations [53, 54]. Many strains, however, were found not to belong to any of the host-specific biotypes and instead were classed as non-host-specific biotypes which are usually associated with several hosts [55]. The use of phenotyping techniques such as multilocus enzyme electrophoresis (MLEE) [56] and later more discriminatory genotyping methods, such as pulsed-field gel electrophoresis (PFGE) [55, 57], multilocus sequence typing (MLST) [56, 58] and whole genome sequencing [59], has clearly demonstrated the existence of specialized host-specific *S. aureus* clones [54].

Microarray studies of animal and human *S. aureus* isolates have shown that strains that are isolated from one host species tend to be uncommon in other species [60], although this delineation is not always absolute [54]. In many respects, the host range of *S. aureus* should be considered an evolving trait [61]. Adaptation to a particular host species does not prevent *S. aureus* strains from causing occasional infections in other species [62]. Wherever there is an interface between different host species, the opportunity exists for bacterial exchange. In most cases, these exchanges lead to transient infections which are short lived due to the failure of the *S. aureus* strain to establish transmission pathways in the new host species [62]. However, sustained interspecies events are known to occur albeit at a lower frequency [62].

A number of independent studies have investigated specific *S. aureus* host-switching events. All of the described host-switch events highlight the significant role that the transfer of MGEs plays in host adaptation and specialization [56, 62, 63]. It is believed that if the conditions under which *S. aureus* host switches occur is understood, then strategies could be developed to curb future host jumps and the emergence of new human pathogens [63].

4. Staphylococcal infections in humans

Infections caused by *S. aureus* are often acute and pyogenic and, if left untreated, may spread to surrounding tissue or via bacteremia to metastatic sites [2]. Some of the most common infections caused by *S. aureus* involve the skin, and include furuncles or boils, cellulitis, impetigo and post-operative wound infections of various sites [2]. Mastitis is one of a variety of skin and soft tissue infections that may be caused by *S. aureus*. Unlike other *S. aureus* infections in humans, staphylococcal mastitis has not been extensively studied [60, 64]. It is estimated that mastitis develops in approximately 1–3% of nursing mothers [65]. Infection usually presents within two to three days after giving birth, with symptoms ranging from cellulitis to abscess formation [65]. In severe cases, systemic symptoms such as fever and chills may arise [65]. *Staphylococcus aureus* may also cause more serious infections such as bacteremia, pneumonia, osteomyelitis, acute endocarditis, myocarditis, pericarditis, cerebritis, meningitis and abscesses of the muscle, urogenital tract, central nervous system and various intra-abdominal organs [2].

Staphylococcal diseases that arise exclusively from the production of staphylococcal toxins include staphylococcal scalded skin syndrome (SSSS), toxic shock syndrome (TSS) and staphylococcal food poisoning [65]. Staphylococcal food poisoning occurs following the ingestion of food contaminated with enterotoxins [66]. Enterotoxins are heat stable and can survive conditions that would ordinarily kill bacteria [67]. Furthermore, enterotoxins are tolerant to low pH conditions and the activity of proteolytic enzymes and are thus able to retain their activity in the digestive tract following ingestion [5, 67]. Following ingestion of contaminated food and a short incubation period (two to eight hours), nausea and vomiting ensue [66]. Diarrhea, hypotension and dehydration may also occur [65]. Staphylococcal food poisoning is usually self-limiting and typically resolves within 24 to 48 hours following the onset of symptoms [3]. Occasionally, the symptoms may be severe enough to warrant hospitalization, particularly in the case of infants, the elderly or immunocompromised individuals [66]. Staphylococcal food poisoning is a common disease but the true incidence is considered to be underestimated due to misdiagnosis, unreported outbreaks, improper specimen collection and laboratory examination [66]. The disease represents a considerable burden in terms of loss of productivity, medical and hospital expenses and financial losses to food industries [66]. Enterotoxin production is not limited to *S. aureus* but has been documented in a number of other staphylococci including *S. hyicus, S. pseudintermedius, S. chromogenes, S. cohnii, S. epidermidis, S. lentus, S. lugdunensis, S. saprophyticus, S. sciuri, S. warneri* and *S. xylosus* [3, 5, 68, 69].

Almost half of all the CNS species that have been identified to date have been implicated in human infections [65]. Coagulase-negative staphylococci, in particular *S. epidermidis*, are frequently responsible for nosocomial infections and prosthetic-device-related infections [27, 70]. The increased infection rate is correlated with increase in the use of prosthetic and indwelling devices in hospitals as well as the larger number of immunocompromised patients [39, 41]. *Staphylococcus epidermidis* is uniquely adapted to colonize prosthetic devices by virtue of the ability of the bacterium to produce an extracellular polysaccharide, also referred to as a glycocalyx or slime layer, which facilitates the formation of a protective biofilm on the surface of the implanted device [39, 65]. The process of biofilm formation and the protective effects conferred upon the bacteria are discussed in further detail below.

Staphylococcus haemolyticus is the second most frequently encountered CNS associated with human infections [2]. *Staphylococcus haemolyticus* has been implicated in native valve endocarditis, septicemia, peritonitis, urinary tract infections and wound and bone and joint infections [2]. *Staphylococcus saprophyticus* is another opportunistic pathogen, which is frequently responsible for causing human urinary tract infections, particularly in young, sexually active females [2, 12].

Two staphylococcal species, *S. lugdunensis* and *S. schleferi,* have been described as emerging zoonotic pathogens [71]. *Staphylococcus lugdunensis,* which is known to cause skin infections and invasive infections, such as endocarditis, osteomyelitis and sepsis in humans, has more recently been described as an animal pathogen implicated in respiratory and skin infections [71, 72]. *Staphylococcus schleiferi,* which has typically been associated with skin infections in pet animals, has also been found associated with endocarditis and metastatic infection as well as endophthalmitis in humans [73, 74]. Both bacterial species have been reported to cause more serious infections than other CNS, but the exact reasons for this enhanced virulence are not known [43, 71].

5. Staphylococcal infections in animals

Amongst all of the described staphylococcal species, only *S. aureus*, *S. epidermidis*, *S. hyicus* and *S. pseudintermedius* are responsible for significant disease conditions in animals [75, 76]. Other *Staphylococcus* spp. are predominantly associated with opportunistic infections in different animal species [75].

In poultry, *S. aureus* is responsible for several infectious conditions including septic arthritis, subdermal abscesses ('bumblefoot'), gangrenous dermatitis and bacterial chrondronecrosis with osteomyelitis [58, 77]. In sheep and goats, *S. aureus* is a common cause of dermatitis whilst in horses and pigs *S. aureus* may cause botryomycosis, a chronic, suppurative granulomatous condition [24]. In companion animals, *S. aureus* causes suppurative conditions similar to those produced by *S. pseudintermedius* [24].

Staphylococcus hyicus is responsible for causing exudative epidermitis in pigs, also known as greasy pig disease, as well as sporadic joint infections and cystitis [24]. In companion animals *S. pseudintermedius* is commonly isolated from cases of pyoderma, otitis externa and other suppurative conditions including mastitis, endometritis, cystitis, osteomyelitis and wound infections [24]. Methicillin-resistant *S. pseudintermedius* is emerging as an important clinical problem in veterinary medicine in many countries [78, 79].

Staphylococcus species can cause intramammary infections in a variety of animal species [24]. Bovine IMIs are the most economically significant, but in areas where sheep and goats are maintained for milking purposes, IMIs caused by staphylococci can cause substantial losses [80]. Similarly, in countries where milk is sourced from buffalo or camels, significant financial losses due to mastitis have been reported [81, 82]. The direct, or obvious, financial losses incurred as a result of IMIs include treatment costs (veterinary fees and drugs); milk that is discarded due to poor quality, or milk lost during the required withdrawal period before and after drug administration; increased labor costs and animal fatalities or euthanasia [83, 84]. In addition to the direct financial losses incurred due to IMIs, a number of indirect costs exist, which are harder to quantify and are often overlooked. Subclinical infections usually proceed

http://dx.doi.org/10.5772/61785

undetected in a herd resulting in a gradual decrease in milk production and a decline in overall milk quality [83]. This leads to a gradual erosion of profit margins, which, even when detected, can take significant time and financial input to rectify [83].

Staphylococcus aureus is possibly the most notorious of all mastitis pathogens by virtue of the fact that infections caused by this species are difficult to treat and tend to become chronic [36]. Coagulase-negative staphylococci are considered to be emerging pathogens, as in many countries the CNS have become the most common bacteria isolated from intramammary infections [9]. The species most commonly isolated from intramammary infections include *S. chromogenes*, *S. epidermidis*, *S. haemolyticus*, *S. simulans* and *S. xylosus* [85, 86].

6. Antimicrobial resistance in staphylococci

Staphylococcus aureus is intrinsically susceptible to all antimicrobials that have been developed [33]. Antimicrobial resistance may be acquired through mutation and selection of resistant bacterial strains or through horizontal transfer of resistance genes from other bacteria of the same or different species [33]. Common mechanisms which are used to circumvent the action of antimicrobials include (i) the production of enzymes that inactivate or destroy the antimicrobial; (ii) a reduction of the bacterial cell wall permeability limiting the antimicrobial access into the cell; (iii) the development of alternative metabolic pathways to those inhibited by the antimicrobial; and (iv) active elimination of the antimicrobial from the bacterial cell or the target site [87, 88]. The mechanisms responsible for antimicrobial resistance in CNS are identical to those occurring in *S. aureus* [89].

6.1. The emergence of resistance in *S. aureus*

Shortly after the introduction of penicillin in human medicine in 1946, reports of *S. aureus* strains exhibiting resistance to this antimicrobial began emerging [90]. Penicillin-resistant staphylococci were first recognized in hospitals and then subsequently in the community [91]. By the late 1960s, more than 80% of both community- and hospital-associated staphylococcal isolates were resistant to penicillin [92]. It is estimated that more than 90% of staphylococcal isolates now produce penicillinase, regardless of the clinical setting [93].

A similar clinical scenario was observed following the introduction of methicillin, the first semisynthetic penicillin resistant to the action of penicillinase [90]. Shortly after the introduction of methicillin in 1959, methicillin-resistant strains were reported [94]. Once again, resistant strains initially presented in the hospital environment; and then by the late 1990s, virulent methicillin-resistant clones emerged in the community [91].

During the 1960s, a number of non-β-lactam antibiotics, such as chloramphenicol, erythromycin, streptomycin and tetracycline, were introduced [89]. Although initially effective against *S. aureus*, resistance to these antimicrobials was eventually observed [89]. By 1976, resistance to gentamicin and kanamycin had been reported, and by the early 1980s, multidrug-resistant *S. aureus* strains were reportedly responsible for nosocomial outbreaks in many countries [47, 95].

Vancomycin and teicoplanin, both glycopeptide antibiotics, have been the frontline treatment for serious methicillin-resistant *Staphylococcus aureus* (MRSA) infections for the last 15 years [47, 96]. Due to the increasing burden of MRSA infections and the concomitant increase in the usage of vancomycin, bacterial isolates showing intermediate susceptibility (not inhibited *in vitro* at concentrations below 4–8 μg/ml, vancomycin-intermediate *S. aureus* (VISA)) were reported in Japan in 1997 [97]. By 2002, vancomycin-resistant *S. aureus* (VRSA; isolates only inhibited at antimicrobial concentrations of 16 μg/ml or more) were encountered in Michigan, United States [33, 98].

A timeline showing the emergence of resistance in *S. aureus* relative to the introduction of significant antimicrobial classes is shown in Figure 2. Several antimicrobials with good anti-staphylococcal activity have been introduced in recent years, including ceftaroline, ceftobiprole, dalbavancin, daptomycin, linezolid, telavancin and tigecycline [99, 100]. Isolates showing reduced susceptibility to daptomycin and resistance to linezolid have already been documented [101]. Undoubtedly, as the use of these drugs becomes more widespread, bacterial resistance will become more common [102].

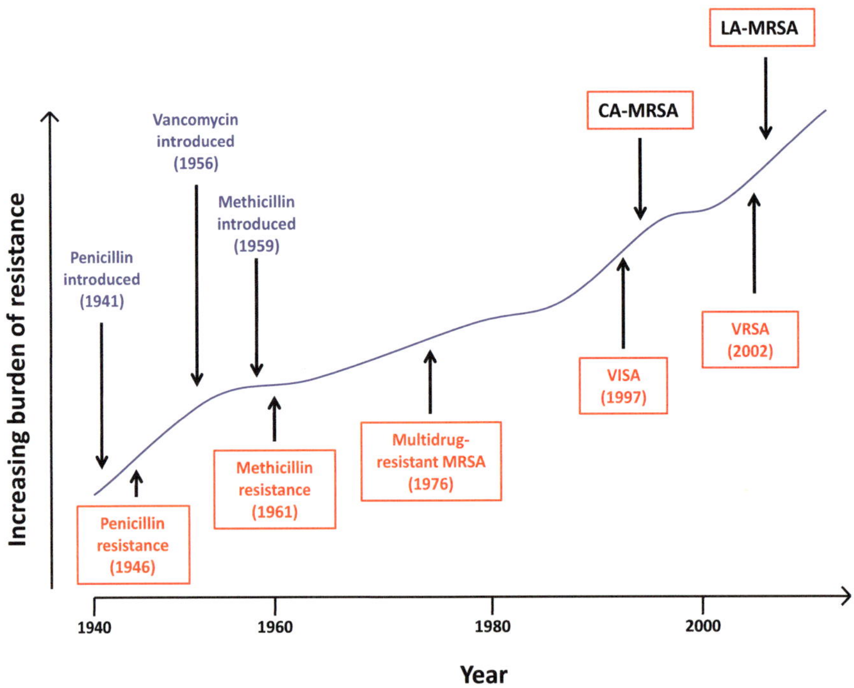

Figure 2. The emergence of antibiotic resistance in *S. aureus* (VISA, vancomycin-intermediate *S. aureus*; VRSA, vancomycin-resistant *S. aureus*; CA-MRSA, community-associated methicillin-resistant *S. aureus*; LA-MRSA, livestock-associated methicillin-resistant *S. aureus*) Adapted from [33, 47].

The distinct lack of novel antimicrobials for future use is a serious cause for concern [93, 103]. Current strategies are aimed at prudent and strategic use of antimicrobials to delay the emergence of resistance and ensure the longevity of antimicrobials in clinical practice [104, 105].

6.2. Mechanism of penicillin resistance in staphylococci

Resistance to penicillin is primarily mediated by the *blaZ* gene, which is responsible for the production of beta-lactamase (penicillinase), an enzyme that hydrolyzes the β-lactam ring of the penicillin molecule [93]. The *blaZ* gene is part of a transposable element located on a large plasmid, which often carries additional antimicrobial resistance genes, which confer resistance to erythromycin, fusidic acid and gentamicin [93]. The plasmid may also carry genes encoding resistance to disinfectants (quaternary ammonium compounds), dyes (acriflavine and ethidium bromide) or heavy metals (cadmium, lead and mercury) [106].

6.3. Mechanism of methicillin resistance in staphylococci

Methicillin resistance arises due to the acquisition of the *mecA* gene, which encodes an alternative penicillin-binding protein, PBP2a (or PBP2'), which has a low affinity for β-lactam antibiotics [14, 100, 107]. The synthesis of PBP2a allows bacterial cell cell wall synthesis to proceed uninterrupted in the presence of β-lactam antibiotics despite the inactivation of the native penicillin-binding protein of the cells [93, 100]. The *mecA* gene confers resistance to all β-lactam antibiotics, including cephalosporins, cefamycins and carbapenems [103, 107].

The *mecA* gene is part of a large mobile genetic element designated the staphylococcal cassette chromosome mec (SCC*mec*) [31, 100]. The SCC*mec* integrates into the staphylococcal chromosome of methicillin-sensitive *S. aureus* at a specific site (*attBscc*) which is located at the 3′ end of an open reading frame of a gene with an unknown function (*orfX*) [33, 108]. In addition to the *mecA* gene, SCC*mec* also carries the genes that control the transcription of the *mecA* gene (*mecI* and *mecR1*) and chromosomal cassette recombinase genes (*ccrA*, *ccrB* or *ccrC*), which mediate the integration and excision of the cassette into the host chromosome [31]. The SCC*mec* element may also contain other genes encoding resistance to antimicrobials, such as aminoglycosides or macrolides and resistance to heavy metal ions [109, 110]. According to their genetic structure and contents, SCC*mec* elements are categorized into several types and subtypes [14, 31]. To date, the website of the International Working Group on the Classification of Staphylococcal Cassette Chromosome elements (IWCC) lists 11 types of SCC*mec* elements (I to XI) [111].

Staphylococcal chromosomal cassettes containing the *mec* gene have been identified not only in *S. aureus* but also in other CPS and CNS [112]. In CNS, SCC*mec* elements exhibit a more polymorphous structure with a larger number of *ccr–mec* combinations being encountered, which have not been described for MRSA [113]. The higher frequency and diversity of SCC*mec* elements in CNS suggest that CNS are a potential reservoir of SCC*mec* elements, which may facilitate and drive the emergence of new MRSA clones [114]. The possible mechanism(s) involved in the horizontal transfer of SCC*mec* elements from CNS to *S. aureus* are currently not known [115].

The origin of the *mecA* gene has been a source of speculation for many years. Homologues of the *mecA* gene have been found in *S. sciuri* and *S. vitulinus*, but in both cases, the *mecA* gene is not located in a *mecA* complex as with SCC*mec* [116]. Tsubakishita and co-workers [108] identified a *mec*A gene homologue in *S. fleuretti*, which shared almost 100% sequence homology with MRSA strain N315 and which resided on a structure almost identical to the *mec*A complex. *Staphylococcus fleuretti* is a member of the *S. sciuri* group of staphylococci and is a commensal bacterium of animals [108]. The occurrence of a direct precursor of the methicillin resistance determinant in a *Staphylococcus* species, which normally resides on animals, suggests that staphylococci of animal origin may be a reservoir for the evolution of novel SCC*mec* elements [116].

Molecular investigations of a *S. aureus* isolate, which was found to be phenotypically resistant to methicillin but negative for the *mec*A gene when tested with a standard diagnostic polymerase chain reaction (PCR) assay, led to the discovery of a novel *mec*A homologue [117]. The *mec*A homologue, initially designated $mecA_{LGA251}$ after *S. aureus* LGA251, the bacterial strain in which the gene was first sequenced, shares 70% nucleotide identity with the conventional *mec*A gene [118]. The work of García-Álvarez and co-workers [117] showed that $mecA_{LGA251}$ was found in *S. aureus* lineages typically associated with cattle, namely clonal complex (CC)130, CC1943 and sequence type (ST)425, suggesting the existence of a zoonotic MRSA reservoir. Furthermore, evidence of animal-to-human transmission of MRSA strains harboring $mecA_{LGA251}$ has been documented [119]. In 2012, the IWCC renamed the *mec*A variant, *mec*C [120]. The *mec*C gene resides on a novel SCC*mec* element designated SCC*mec* XI [121]. Methicillin-resistant *S. aureus* strains carrying the *mec*C gene have been shown to cause a range of infections in humans and appear to be predominantly community associated [118, 119]. The prevalence of *mec*C in CNS has not been extensively explored as yet [60], but an allotype of the *mec*C gene has been detected in a *S. xylosus* strain [118].

6.3.1. Healthcare-associated MRSA

Traditionally, MRSA has been considered a hospital- or healthcare-associated pathogen (HA-MRSA) primarily infecting people who are immunocompromised or who have had surgery or medical device implants [122, 123]. Healthcare-associated MRSA strains usually carry SCC*mec* types I, II and III and are multidrug resistant [14]. Worldwide, the majority of HA-MRSA strains belong to CC5, CC8, CC22, CC30 and CC45 [14, 122].

6.3.2. Community-associated MRSA

Since the mid-1990s, MRSA strains were increasingly reported in healthy people without any healthcare-associated risk factors [31, 122]. These cases were termed community-associated MRSA (CA-MRSA), and genetic analyses revealed that these *S. aureus* isolates were genetically distinct from the typical HA-MRSA strains [31]. Community-associated MRSA strains are primarily associated with SCC*mec* types IV and V, which typically lack non-β-lactam resistance genes [124]. Most CA-MRSA strains belong to sequence type (ST)1, ST8, ST30, ST59, ST80 and ST93 [14, 122] with ST8 ('USA300') being the most common clonal lineage in the USA and ST80 the most common in Europe [125, 126]. Carriage of the gene encoding the Panton–Valentine leukocidin appears to be epidemiologically associated with certain CA-MRSA strains [14, 123].

6.3.3. Livestock-associated MRSA

The emergence of a third group of MRSA strains was witnessed in the last decade, which was described following investigations that began on a pig farm in the Netherlands [54, 127]. Pig farmers and other close human contacts were found to be at a higher risk of carrying MRSA than members of the population who did not frequent pig farms [128]. This group of MRSA strains, initially referred to as 'non-typeable MRSA' or 'pig MRSA', was found to belong to a single clonal complex, CC398, with the majority of strains belonging to sequence type (ST)398 [31]. Methicillin-resistant *S. aureus* ST398 has subsequently been isolated from other animal species, including dogs, horses, veal calves and poultry [125, 129–131], and it has therefore been designated livestock-associated MRSA (LA-MRSA) [125]. It has been shown that persons in direct (occupational) contact with LA-MRSA-positive animals, such as farmers, laborers, veterinarians and abattoir staff, have an increased risk of becoming MRSA carriers [31]. Methicillin-resistant *S. aureus* ST398 strains can cause infections in both animals [31] and humans [117]. Furthermore, certain strains belonging to an independent clade within CC398 have been associated with direct human-to-human transmission without prior exposure to livestock [132].

Livestock-associated MRSA ST398 carries SCC*mec* element IV or V [133]. These strains are generally resistant to tetracycline while resistance to aminoglycosides, lincosamides, macrolides and trimethoprim has also been documented [31]. Fluoroquinolone resistance has also been reported in isolates from Germany [14]. The LA-MRSA ST398 strains have been found to carry previously unidentified resistance genes, such as *dfr*K, a novel, plasmid-borne trimethoprim resistance gene [134]. This gene is located close to *tet*L, which would allow for the selection of either gene by the use of tetracycline or trimethoprim, both of which are used in veterinary medicine [135]. A novel ABC efflux pump encoding gene, *vga*C, which confers resistance to lincosamides and streptogramins, was also found on the same plasmid [134]. The multidrug resistance gene, *cfr*, was found in two porcine *S. aureus* isolates from Germany, one MRSA ST398 and one MSSA ST9 [136]. The *cfr* gene confers resistance to a number of antimicrobials including lincosamides, oxazolidinones, phenicols pleuromutilins and streptogramin A [133].

Molecular typing and whole genome sequencing have revealed that LA-MRSA CC398 strains originated from human-methicillin-sensitive *S. aureus* strains, which crossed the species barrier and in the process lost phage-carrying virulence genes that are usually found in human isolates [137]. The host switch from humans to livestock was further accompanied by the acquisition of methicillin and tetracycline resistance genes [137], suggesting that an antibiotic selective pressure exists in the livestock industry [138].

6.4. Mechanisms of vancomycin resistance in staphylococci

The molecular mechanisms underlying VISA and VRSA are different [139, 140]. Intermediate vancomycin resistance is associated with the presence of a thickened and/or poorly cross-linked peptidoglycan bacterial cell wall [140]. The altered cell wall structure traps the antimicrobial molecules reducing cellular penetration and preventing the antimicrobial from reaching its target site [140]. Heteroresistant VISA isolates (hVISA) have been described by

Hiramatsu and co-workers [141]. Heteroresistant strains are susceptible to vancomycin but contain a small subpopulation of cells, approximately one in every 10^6 cells, which exhibit resistance. It is proposed that hVISA may be a precursor to VISA and, as such, needs to be detected so that appropriate control measures can be implemented to limit the spread of the bacterium [142].

Vancomycin-resistant *S. aureus* strains do not arise from VISA but have acquired the complete genetic apparatus mediating resistance to glycopeptides from vancomycin-resistant enterococci [51, 93, 98]. The genes encoding vancomycin resistance, collectively referred to as the *van*A gene complex, reside on a transposon, Tn*1546* [139]. The transposon is carried by a conjugative plasmid and is transmissible to a number of Gram-positive bacterial genera including *Bacillus*, *Staphylococcus* and *Streptococcus* [139].

7. Alternate bacterial strategies to circumvent the action of antimicrobials

In addition to the challenges posed by antimicrobial resistance, the treatment of staphylococcal infections is further complicated by a number of strategies that staphylococci have developed, which enable the bacteria to evade the host immune response and the activity of antimicrobials [12, 143]. Two strategies, namely the formation of biofilms and the development of small-colony variants, will be discussed in further detail.

7.1. The formation of biofilms

Biofilms can be described as large, amorphous aggregates of bacterial cells encased in extracellular material comprising *inter alia,* bacterial by-products, polysaccharides and proteins [12]. Biofilms may form on abiotic surfaces, such as implanted medical devices as well as biotic surfaces, such as host tissue [12, 39]. The formation of biofilms can be visualized as being a four-step process: (i) the attachment of bacteria to the surface; (ii) proliferation of the bacterial cells; (iii) biofilm growth and maturation; and finally (iv) dissociation and dissemination of bacterial cells to new sites [12, 39].

The formation of biofilms affords bacterial cell protection from a multitude of chemical, cellular and physical antagonists [143]. The bacteria encased in biofilms are able to tolerate significantly higher concentrations of antimicrobials and disinfectants than free-floating bacterial cells [39, 143, 144]. Furthermore, the bacterial cells residing in biofilms are more resistant to phagocytosis and are protected from pH extremes and physical desiccation [143]. The protective effect of biofilms is in part attributable to the physiological changes that the bacterial cells undergo whilst growing *en masse*. Bacteria existing within biofilms grow more slowly than exponential-phase bacteria [143]. This is partly due to restricted diffusion of gases and nutrients within the biofilm environment, but this is also affected by alterations in bacterial gene expression [145]. Beenken and co-workers [145] revealed a change in the expression of 580 genes (more than 20% of the genome) when using microarrays to study differences between *S. aureus* cells growing in biofilm and planktonic cultures.

The close contact between bacterial cells residing in biofilm communities facilitates and promotes the exchange of MGEs [146]. The horizontal transfer of plasmids in biofilms is typically higher than observed between cells existing in a planktonic state and, in fact, studies have shown that biofilms promote plasmid stability and may enhance the host range of MGEs [146]. As previously discussed, the exchange of MGEs plays a significant role in the emergence of new, potentially more virulent, staphylococcal strains.

7.2. Intracellular persistence and the formation of small-colony variants

The ability of staphylococci to persist intracellularly in non-professional phagocyctic cells following ingestion affords protection to the bacteria from the host immune system as well as the action of antimicrobials [12]. The adaptation to an intracellular environment is accompanied by the formation of 'small-colony variants' (SCVs), which represent an alternate phenotypic and metabolic state of the normal, wild-type, staphylococcal phenotype [12, 147]. The SCV phenotype is characterized by a reduced growth rate as well as substantial changes in gene expression [12]. The altered phenotypic state also affects the susceptibility of the bacteria to antimicrobials [144]. In addition to phagocytes, internalization of *S. epidermidis* in human endothelial cells and bone cells has been demonstrated [12].

The formation of biofilms and small-colony variants is implicated in persistent and relapsing infections, and, as such, it poses a significant challenge for the treatment staphylococcal infections [12, 147].

8. Use of antimicrobials in animal health and food animal production operations and implications for human health

Antimicrobials are used in animal health and food production to treat and prevent disease and, more contentiously, for growth promotion in food production animals [148, 149]. The volume of antimicrobials used in animals is larger than the volumes used in human medicine even in countries where strict regulations regarding antimicrobials are enforced [148]. Exact data on antimicrobial consumption in animals are scarce and only available for a few countries [148]. Recent data from the USA suggest that almost 80% of antimicrobials produced are used in food-producing animal operations [150–152] and 70% hereof are used for non-therapeutic purposes [153, 154]. The largest users of antimicrobials are typically the poultry and swine producers due to the intensive nature of these production systems [155].

The use and administration of antimicrobials in companion animals (cats, dogs and horses) fall largely under the control of veterinary practitioners [148, 156]. Individual animals are examined and diagnosed, following which the appropriate therapeutic recourse is selected [148, 156]. In the event that antimicrobials are administered, this is done in accordance with the manufacturer's recommendations ensuring the prudent use of antimicrobials [148]. In contrast, the use of antimicrobials in food production animals (livestock and poultry) is often done with little or no veterinary consultation [148]. Many antimicrobials are accessible to producers as 'over-the-counter' remedies from local retailers, thereby limiting the control over the use of these products [148, 157]. In food production animals, antimicrobials may be applied therapeutically to treat sick individuals, but it is more common for producers to apply antimicrobials to entire herds or flocks in order to treat sick animals and to curb the spread of infectious organisms to healthy animals [148, 156]. The administration of antimicrobials in this manner is termed metaphylaxis [148, 158].

In food production systems, antimicrobials are often intentionally administered to animals in sub-therapeutic doses to promote growth and enhance feed efficiency [148]. The benefits of using antimicrobials as 'growth promoters' were recognized as early as the 1940s [149, 158]. Researchers observed that poultry that were administered vitamin B12 in the form of crude *Streptococcus aureofaciens* fermentations showed improved growth compared to birds given purified vitamin B12 [159]. It was speculated that the crude fermentations contained an unidentified growth factor, which enhanced growth [158]. The growth factor in the fermentation product was subsequently identified as chlortetracycline [158]. Shortly after this observation, the US Food and Drug Administration (FDA) approved the inclusion of certain antimicrobials into animal feed to enhance animal growth and production as well as prevent disease [158]. Some of the antimicrobials which have been utilized as growth promoters in some countries include: avilamycin (everninomycin), avoparcin (glycopeptide), bacitracin (polypeptide), bambermycin (glycolipid), carbadox and olaquindox (quinoxalines), lincomycin (lincosamides), pencillin (β-lactams), streptomycin (aminoglycosides), tetracycline and chlortetracycline (tetracyclines), tylosin and spiramycin (macrolides) and virginiamycin (streptogramin) [156, 159, 160].

The use of antimicrobials in animals, particularly as growth promoters in food producing animals, has been subjected to intense scrutiny and is frequently criticized as a driving force behind the emergence, maintenance and horizontal transfer of antimicrobial-resistant determinants in bacteria [161, 162]. The principle concern is the potential zoonotic transmission of antimicrobial-resistant pathogenic and non-pathogenic bacteria to humans either through direct contact with animals or indirectly through contact with the animals' environment or through the food chain [161, 163]. Due to public concerns and increasing scientific evidence, stricter regulations regarding the use of growth promoters have been implemented [164]. The European Union began phasing out the use of antimicrobials for growth promotion in the late 1990s [163]. By the year 2000, Denmark had successfully implemented a complete ban of antimicrobial growth promoters in food animal production [157, 160]. Stakeholders in favor of restrictions have argued that in countries like Denmark, where bans have been introduced, there has been a concomitant decrease in antimicrobial resistance in animal and human bacterial isolates [164]. Opponents to the ban of growth promoters have, however, questioned the evidence provided by supporters of the ban and have argued that a decline in the use of growth promoters will negatively affect productivity and animal health, which will in turn lead to an increase in the therapeutic use of antimicrobials [149, 164]. A number of excellent reviews have examined the complexity and debate surrounding the use of growth promoters in livestock production, and the reader is referred to these texts for further information [148, 149, 157, 165–167].

9. The interface between human and animal populations

The dynamics of staphylococcal antimicrobial resistance and bacterial transmission at the human–animal interface will be considered separately for companion animals (cats, dogs and horses) and food production animals (livestock and poultry). Consideration will also be given to the intersection of humans and animal carcasses further along the food chain in the abattoir.

9.1. Companion animals

It is common in developed countries for humans to own companion animals [126]. Due to the close contact between humans and their pets, the opportunity for the transmission of bacteria between hosts is high [126]. Numerous reports have documented the transmission of MRSA strains between humans and dogs [168–174], humans and cats [175, 176] and humans and horses [177, 178]. Bacterial transmission of MRSA leads to both hosts becoming colonized, which places the hosts at a higher risk of being infected by the colonizing strain when the opportunity presents [78]. Furthermore, the colonized hosts serve as reservoirs of MRSA for other members of the household [179, 180].

Molecular genotyping of MRSA isolates recovered from companion animals has revealed that the *S. aureus* strains recovered from colonized and infected animals usually belong to clonal complexes implicated in human infections [126, 171, 173, 174, 177, 181, 182]. An investigation conducted in the United Kingdom examined the occurrence and the genetic relatedness of MRSA recovered from veterinary personnel and hospitalized animals in a small animal hospital [171]. Eighty-two percent (23/28) of the MRSA isolates recovered from the nasal mucosa of staff, hospitalized dogs and the environment were genetically related to EMRSA-15 (ST22), the predominant MRSA clone responsible for nosocomial infections in the United Kingdom [171]. In the USA, the most common MRSA clone recovered from companion animals is the ST5 clone, which is also the most common HA-MRSA clone in humans [171]. These data have suggested that the transmission of MRSA usually occurs from the human host to their respective pet [78, 179].

In general, prevalence studies seem to suggest that MRSA colonization amongst healthy pets is low [126, 176]. Higher MRSA colonization rates have been documented amongst companion animals in settings like animal shelters and veterinary hospitals [126, 171, 183]. Presumably, due to the relatively low MRSA colonization of companion animals there is currently no significant evidence indicating that pet owners are at an increased risk of MRSA colonization or infection compared with humans who do not own pets [107]. However, it is suggested that the lack of evidence may be partly attributed to the paucity of studies examining this particular aspect of animal ownership [107].

Since 2006, there has been a significant increase in the number of documented cases involving the isolation of methicillin-resistant *S. pseudintermedius* (MRSP) strains from surgical wound infections of dogs and cats [79]. A few studies have reported the occurrence of indistinguishable strains of MRSP from humans and their canine companions [176] and amongst animals and workers in veterinary clinics [184]. In Japan, a study investigating the prevalence of MRSP in a veterinary teaching hospital, cultured MRSP from 17 dogs and a staff member [25]. The isolate recovered from the employee had an antimicrobial susceptibility pattern and a PFGE profile similar to isolates recovered from dogs handled at the facility, indicating zoonotic transmission [25]. A study investigating the prevalence of MRSP in staff working at a veterinary dermatology practice reported that 5.3% (9/171) of the staff tested positive [185]. In general, owners of infected pets and veterinarians handling infected animals seem to have a higher risk of being MRSP positive [79]. In all documented cases, MRSP-positive individuals have been asymptomatic [79].

9.2. Food production animals

Livestock and poultry production has, over the past few decades, intensified in order to keep abreast with the food demands posed by a burgeoning human population [138, 148]. Larger numbers of animals are maintained under confined conditions in order to maximize productivity and improve profit margins. Accompanying these changes in farming practices has been an increase in the use of antimicrobials as well as increase in the proximity in which animals and humans co-exist [137, 138]. The close proximity of animal and human hosts has in turn increased opportunities for the transmission and exchange of microbial flora [56, 138]. It is well established that individuals such as farmers, veterinarians, farm laborers and abattoir workers working in close contact with animals have a greater risk of being colonized or even infected with zoonotic bacteria carried by animals than individuals that do not interact with animals [31]. The relatively recent description of zoonotic LA-MRSA ST398 and the novel methicillin resistance gene, *mec*C, has once again highlighted the implications associated with the horizontal transmission of pathogenic bacteria between animal and human hosts and the role of animals in the epidemiology and the evolution of human disease [118, 186].

Since the description of LA-MRSA, a plethora of studies have been conducted to estimate the prevalence of MRSA in different food animals, and a number of reviews have been published [14, 31, 107, 125]. Livestock-associated MRSA has been extensively described in pig production systems with many investigations documenting the transmission of CC398 between animals and close human contacts [187–193]. A study conducted in Germany found 86% (97/113) of people who worked with pigs to be asymptomatic carriers of CC398 MRSA [190]. Interestingly, in the same study, sampling of the family members of CC398 MRSA carriers showed that 4.3% (5/116) of these individuals, who had no direct exposure to pigs, were colonized by the same MRSA strain [190]. Nasal colonization was also found in 45% (22/49) of veterinarians frequenting pig farms in the study area and in 9% (4/44) of their family members who had not been exposed to pigs [190]. A pilot study conducted in two large pig production systems in the USA revealed an overall MRSA prevalence of 49% (147/299) in the animals sampled and 45% (9/20) of the farm workers [194]. All MRSA isolates belonged to ST398 [194]. In Belgium, 37.8% (48/129) of close human contacts sampled from 50 pig farms were found to be colonized by MRSA ST398 [191]. An identical MRSA strain was recovered from the skin lesions of one worker who was sampled at the time of the study [191]. In some geographical settings, other MRSA clones have been found to colonize pigs. In China, MRSA strains belonging to ST9 were commonly isolated from pigs and close human contacts [195, 196]. In Italy, pigs sampled at abattoirs were found to be colonized by MRSA ST9, ST(CC)97 and ST398 [197]. Further, the presence of human-associated CA-MRSA t127, ST1 and SCC*mec* type V was detected [197]. Despite the high rate of LA-MRSA colonization in pigs, this *S. aureus* clone has only been implicated in sporadic clinical infections in pigs [107]. Livestock-associated MRSA has been isolated from skin infections such as exudative epidermidis and infections of the urogenital tract and the uterus and mammary gland of pigs [14].

In the Netherlands, MRSA ST398 colonization has been documented in veal calves and close human contacts [131]. From the 102 farms sampled in one study, MRSA was isolated from animals on 88% (90/102) of the farms investigated [131]. Overall, 28% (602/2151) of the animals and 33% (32/97) of the farmers sampled tested positive for MRSA [131]. The MRSA strains recovered from the human and animal samples included ST398 as well as ST5, ST15, ST45 and CC34 from the human specimens and ST97, ST239, ST1159 and CC425 from the calves [131]. The data clearly demonstrated that MRSA colonization of human contacts was strongly associated with the intensity of animal contact and with the number of MRSA-positive animals on the farm [131]. Furthermore, a direct correlation was observed between MRSA prevalence and farm hygiene practices [131].

In dairy cattle operations, LA-MRSA ST398 has been isolated from clinical and subclinical milk samples. One of the first reports, emanating from Belgium, recovered LA-MRSA from 9.3% (11/118) of the dairy farms surveyed [198]. The prevalence on positive farms varied between 3.9% and 7.4% [198]. Methicillin-resistant *S. aureus* ST398 has also been reported from dairy herds in Germany [199] and Switzerland [61, 200]. Juhász-Kaszanyitzky and co-workers [201] published the first report documenting the transmission of MRSA between dairy cows with mastitis and a close contact worker on the farm. In this study, identical MRSA strains, belonging to MLST ST1, were recovered from both animal and human hosts. The direction of transmission, from bovine to human or human to bovine could, however, not be established [201].

One of the first reports of LA-MRSA in poultry emerged following a study conducted in Belgium [130]. The researchers reported that 12% (10/81) of the *S. aureus* isolates recovered from the nasal and cloacal swabs of healthy broiler chickens belonged to *spa* types associated with CC398 [130]. A further study in Belgium identified a new *spa* type, t1456, within CC398 following a random sampling of broiler farms [202]. Despite sporadic reports on the isolation of CC398 from poultry operations, the epidemiology of LA-MRSA in poultry is still unclear [14].

According to Schwabe [203], a zoonosis is described as a 'shared infection' of animals and man, without ascribing direction of transmission from one host to the other. Inasmuch as bacterial transfer and colonization, or infection, of humans are of significant concern to human medicine, the reverse scenario, which is often overlooked, warrants consideration. Humans may represent an important source of new bacterial strains, which can cause disease in livestock and, as such, pose a potential threat to food security [138]. Several molecular genotyping studies, which have traced the origins of epidemic *S. aureus* clones in human and animal hosts, have reported that the majority of host-switch events have involved the movement and adaptation of bacteria from human to animal hosts [62]. Both

LA-MRSA ST398 and the major pathogenic *S. aureus* ST5 clone, responsible for lameness in poultry, have been shown to originate from humans but have now adapted and diversified to spread in animal hosts [58, 137].

Irrespective of the direction of bacterial transmission, it is of mutual benefit to both human and animal health that bacterial populations at the interface between different host species are monitored. Surveillance is therefore advocated in order to monitor changes in the epidemiology and virulence of bacterial strains and to enable appropriate pre-emptive measures to be taken [138].

9.3. Food animal products

The abattoir environment presents a dynamic interface between humans and animals largely due to the fact that abattoirs process large numbers of animals originating from different farms across a relatively broad geographic expanse. During slaughtering and subsequent processing, it is quite plausible for carcasses to become contaminated with staphylococcal strains originating from animals, abattoir workers or the environment [14]. Numerous reports have documented the occurrence of CA-MRSA, HA-MRSA and LA-MRSA strains from different meat products [14, 204, 205, 206]. An extensive study conducted in the Netherlands demonstrated the presence of LA-MRSA on a variety of raw meat products collected from retail outlets [204]. In this study, 11.9% (264/2217) of the raw meat products analyzed were found to be positive for MRSA [204]. It was further shown that 85% (224/264) of the MRSA strains belonged to *spa* types associated with CC398 [204]. A survey conducted in the USA found 39.2% (47/120) of the retail meat samples analyzed to be positive for *S. aureus*. Five percent (6/120) of the *S. aureus* isolates were resistant to methicillin. Molecular typing identified the isolates as belonging to the ST5 and ST8 lineages [205]. A similar survey conducted in Canada found 7.7% (31/402) of the meat samples analyzed contained MRSA [206, 207]. The three major sequence types obtained were ST5 (29%), ST8 (39%) and ST398 (32%) [206, 207].

The principal concern arising from the presence of MRSA in food is the development of food poisoning following ingestion of preformed staphylococcal enterotoxins [207]. The best preventative measure is to ensure the correct handling and storage of food to reduce the risk of enterotoxins being produced [207]. Another concern regarding the presence of MRSA on meat is that people may become colonized or infected from handling or eating contaminated meat [205, 207]. Regarding the latter, there is, at present, no substantial data to support or refute this concern. More intensive surveillance is needed to elucidate the true role of food contamination in the development of human diseases [107].

10. Monitoring antimicrobial resistance in staphylococci at the human–animal interface

In addition to direct contact between animal and human hosts, the transmission of antimicrobial-resistant bacteria and resistance genes may occur through a number of routes [76, 149].

http://dx.doi.org/10.5772/61785

Figure 3 presents some of the potential routes of bacterial transmission taking into consideration the role of the environment as well as aspects related to the movement of animals, food products and human contacts. The globalized trade of live animals and/or meat products is one of the features of modern food production systems, which has the potential to elaborate the impact of antimicrobial-resistant bacteria of animal origin [138].

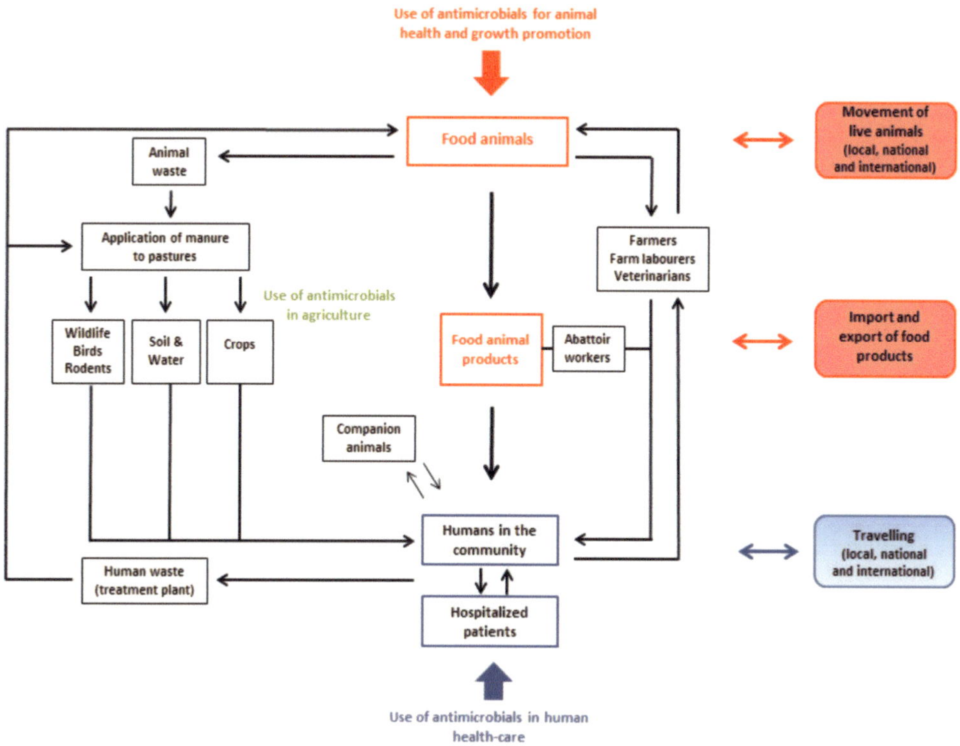

Figure 3. Potential routes of dissemination of antimicrobial-resistant bacteria and antimicrobial resistance genes [76, 149]. ©2005 American Society for Microbiology. Adapted with permission. No further reproduction or distribution is permitted without the prior written permission of American Society for Microbiology

In order to be able to accurately assess the impact of antimicrobial use in animal health and food production operations on human medicine, integrated surveillance programmes are needed [148]. The formulation and implementation of surveillance programmes require a concerted effort from role-players in multiple disciplines. Funding, infrastructure, political 'buy-in' and the support of several role-players are key to the success of these programs [148]. Currently, only a few countries have been able to implement successful monitoring programmes [148]. One of the longest running and most successful programmes is the Danish Integrated Antimicrobial Resistance Monitoring and Research Programme (DANMAP), which has been systematically collecting and analyzing data since 1995 [163]. The programme utilizes a 'one-health' approach and entails the monitoring of the entire food chain from 'farm to fork to sickbed' [208]. The objectives of DANMAP are summarized as follows:

- to monitor the use of antimicrobial agents in food animals and humans;
- to monitor the occurrence of antimicrobial resistance in bacteria isolated from food animals, food of animal origin and humans;
- to study associations between antimicrobial consumption and antimicrobial resistance; and
- to identify routes of transmission of resistant bacteria and/or resistance determinants and areas for further research [163, 208].

Results from DANMAP are reported annually and are accessible online [163]. The data accumulated from long-term surveillance programmes should enable resistance trends to be monitored over periods of time as well as identify emerging problems so that adequate intervention strategies can be implemented [148, 208].

In accordance with Office International des Epizooties (OIE) guidelines, surveillance programmes should investigate antimicrobial resistance in the following groups of bacteria:

1. Human and animal pathogens that cause infections. These bacteria are thought to reflect resistance caused by the use of antimicrobials in the respective reservoirs.
2. Zoonotic bacteria that can develop resistance in the animal reservoir and which can be transmitted to humans via direct contact or consumption of contaminated food. These bacteria may subsequently compromise treatment when causing infection in humans.
3. Sentinel or indicator bacteria, such as enterococci and *Escherichia coli,* are selected for monitoring purposes due to their ubiquity in animals, foods and humans. Furthermore, these bacteria readily develop or transfer antimicrobial resistance in response to selective pressure in both human and animals and are considered reservoirs of resistance determinants [148, 208, 209].

The staphylococci of animal origin which are commonly monitored as part of surveillance programmes include *S. aureus* and coagulase-negative staphylococci from bovine mastitis cases as well as *S. hyicus* isolates from cases of exudative epidermitis in pigs [148, 163]. From human health laboratories, *S. aureus* isolates derived from blood, urine and CSF samples are used for surveillance purposes [208, 209]. Some surveillance programmes, such as the British Society for Antimicrobial Chemotherapy Resistance Surveillance project, extend monitoring to include CNS species [209].

11. Evaluating the antimicrobial susceptibility of staphylococcal isolates

In a clinical context, evaluating the antimicrobial susceptibility of bacterial isolates is an important aid for practitioners needing to make decisions regarding the appropriate therapeutic treatment of infected patients [88]. Antimicrobial susceptibility testing of bacterial isolates also provides essential data for surveillance programs as previously discussed. Several methodologies exist for evaluating the *in vitro* susceptibility of bacterial isolates to different classes of antimicrobials. The two principal methods used are agar disk diffusion and the broth micro-dilution minimum inhibitory concentration (MIC) method [148, 210]. The agar disk diffusion method provides qualitative results that categorize isolates as susceptible, intermediate or resistant to the antimicrobial(s) under evaluation [135, 210]. The method is relatively cost-effective and flexible with respect to the panel of antimicrobials that can be selected for testing [135]. The MIC method may be performed in a variety of formats ranging from in-house prepared plates or broths to commercially available micro-dilution plates or gradient strips [210]. The MIC method provides a quantitative result expressed in micrograms per milliliter as well as a categorization of the bacterium as susceptible or resistant [135, 210]. Since the method is able to quantify antimicrobial susceptibility, the MIC is the preferred method for use in surveillance or epidemiological programs [148].

Irrespective of the test methodology selected, it is imperative that all antimicrobial susceptibility tests are conducted in accordance with the international standard being followed, namely the Clinical Laboratory Standards Institute (CLSI), the European Committee on Antimicrobial Susceptibility Testing (EUCAST) or other recognized national standards [210]. Furthermore, it should be ensured that all of the appropriate quality control measures advocated by the standard are implemented and rigorously followed [210].

In vitro methods for analyzing the antimicrobial susceptibility do not take into consideration the protective effect afforded by biofilm growth, which commonly occurs during the course of staphylococcal infections [143]. Due to the protective environment afforded by biofilm growth and the accompanying changes in bacterial physiology, bacterial cells growing in biofilms are typically able to tolerate antimicrobial concentrations 10-fold to 1000-fold higher than planktonic bacterial populations [143]. A few methods have evolved to investigate the antimicrobial susceptibility of isolates growing in biofilms, with the commercially available method from Innovotech Inc. (Edmonton, Canada) gaining wide acceptance. The Innovotech MBEC™ P&G system is a uniquely designed microtiter plate with 96 identical pegs protruding from the plastic lid (Innovotech Inc., 2012). The system facilitates the generation of 96 identical biofilms on the pegs which can be subjected to varying concentrations of antimicrobial or disinfectant to calculate the minimum biofilm eradication concentration (MBEC) and MIC values for each test isolate (Innovotech Inc., 2012). The Innovotech MBEC™ P&G system (formerly called the Calgary biofilm device) has been used in a number of applications to examine the effect of different chemicals on staphylococcal biofilms [211–215].

11.1. Detection of antimicrobial resistance genes in staphylococcal isolates

A complementary approach to phenotypically evaluating the susceptibility of staphylococcal isolates is to screen test isolates for specific antimicrobial resistance genes using molecular assays, such as PCR and real-time PCR [24, 216]. This approach is still only infrequently used in routine clinical diagnostic work, but from a research perspective, molecular screening has provided a wealth of information with respect to the distribution and spread of resistance genes amongst bacteria [88].

An obstacle to using DNA-based assays for resistance testing is the formidable complexity of resistance mechanisms that exist [217]. It is common for resistance to an antimicrobial to involve multiple genes and, in some cases, not all of the mechanisms involved have been identified [217]. The use of microarrays is one manner in which this limitation has been overcome [216]. Microarray analysis enables bacterial isolates to be simultaneously screened for a large number of gene targets [216]. A DNA microarray consists of an orderly arrangement of DNA probes which have been spotted onto a solid support, such as a silicon chip, glass slide or nylon membrane [216]. Bacterial DNA or cDNA is labelled with a fluorescent dye and allowed to hybridize to the microarray [216]. One of the microarrays currently available commercially, the StaphyType Kit (Alere Technologies, Jena, Germany) permits the simultaneous screening of 334 *S. aureus* gene targets. In addition to screening for a multitude of antimicrobial resistance genes, the kit screens bacterial isolates for species-specific gene markers, toxin-encoding genes and genes encoding specific tissue-binding proteins [218].

12. Epidemiological molecular typing systems for staphylococci

Bacterial typing is important for both clinical and epidemiological investigations to determine the source(s) of infection, routes of transmission in disease outbreaks or the analysis of the genetic relatedness or specific characteristics of bacterial strains [219]. A number of different typing techniques have been developed, each with specific advantages and drawbacks. It is therefore imperative that the most appropriate method, or combination of methods, be selected depending on the purpose of the investigation on hand [219].

Pulsed-field gel electrophoresis is a highly discriminatory technique and is considered to be the 'gold standard' for typing *S. aureus* isolates of both human and animal origin [14]. Pulsed-field gel electrophoresis is also the recommended strain typing technique for *S. epidermidis* and other CNS [220]. Pulsed-field gel electrophoresis detects rapidly accumulating genetic variation and is therefore useful for distinguishing strains for the investigation of an outbreak or for examining the phylogeny of a small bacterial population [60]. The PFGE technique is based on the digestion of bacterial DNA with restriction enzymes that cleave specific recognition sites along the chromosome [221]. The restriction enzyme digestion generates a number of DNA fragments, which are resolved by electrophoresis in an electric field, which is pulsed at different angles across the gel. The resulting banding patterns are analyzed using specific software and interpretations made according to the criteria of Tenover and co-workers [222]. The principal drawbacks of this technique are the fact that this method is technically demanding and time consuming and requires several days before results are available [223]. Furthermore, specialized equipment is required to perform the gel electrophoresis [122, 223]. Interlaboratory reproducibility of results has also been problematic, making the comparison of data generated by different laboratories quite difficult [122].

Multilocus sequence typing (MLST) is a sequence-based genotyping method, which is performed by sequence analysis of approximately 450-bp internal fragments of seven housekeeping genes [224]. The DNA sequences for each locus are assigned distinct allele identification numbers, and the combination of the numbers defined for all loci is used to generate the sequence type (ST) [33, 122]. Isolates that have identical sequences at all seven loci are considered a clone, whereas sequence types that differ by single nucleotide polymorphisms at fewer than three loci are considered closely related and are grouped in clonal complexes (CC) [14, 33]. In contrast to PFGE, MLST indexes genetic variations that accumulate slowly over time [125]. Multilocus sequence typing is, therefore, better suited to measure evolutionary changes over a relatively long time span and is the best method for studying the global epidemiology and frequency of specific bacterial lineages [60, 125]. The method is highly discriminatory and has the distinct advantage of enabling results from other laboratories and studies to be compared using the Internet [122, 224]. At present, the greatest limitation to using MLST is the high cost associated with the sequencing of multiple gene loci [125].

Typing of the *spa* gene is also widely used for the epidemiological study of *S. aureus* isolates [1]. The *spa* gene encodes protein A, an important virulence factor of *S. aureus* [225]. The typing method entails the DNA amplification and sequencing of a polymorphic 24-bp variable-number tandem repeat (VNTR) within the coding region of the *spa* gene followed by the assessment of the data using a central online server. Typing of the *spa* gene has been found to be a suitable typing method for conducting both local and global epidemiological studies [226]. This method has been found to have a greater discriminatory power than MLST but it is less discriminatory than PFGE [122, 227, 228]. Since *spa* typing involves the sequencing of only a single locus compared with MLST, it is cheaper, less laborious and less time consuming to perform [125, 228]. A potential problem, however, is that unrelated lineages can sometimes contain similar *spa* types [125].

Typing of the SCC*mec* element is one of the most important epidemiological tools for studying methicillin-resistant staphylococci [228]. A number of multiplex PCR and real-time PCR assays have been developed to classify the different SCC*mec* types and subtypes [229–234]. An overview of the scope and drawback of various SCC*mec* typing methods, which have been developed, can be found elsewhere [91]. At present, there is no universally accepted assay which can identify and differentiate all of the *mec* types and subtypes [122]. Furthermore, since the described PCR assays target different regions of the SCC*mec* element, it is not uncommon for discrepant results to be obtained when different methods are used to test the same isolates [228].

13. Concluding remarks

Staphylococci are ubiquitous in the environment and occur commensally on the skin and mucous membranes of humans and animal hosts. The genetic flexibility of bacteria in this genus, particular *S. aureus*, is the primary evolutionary driving force behind the emergence of new strains exhibiting enhanced virulence and antimicrobial resistance. The use of antimicrobials in animal health and food animal production operations has been implicated as a driving force behind the development of antimicrobial-resistant bacteria, which can transfer to humans through direct contact or indirectly through the food chain or environment. However, much of the evidence put forward to corroborate the argument against the use of antimicrobials in food animal production operations is tenuous and, if anything, it supports the need for further surveillance data. The implementation and maintenance of national and international integrated antimicrobial resistance surveillance systems are required. Through active monitoring, potential problems can be identified and appropriate guidelines and policies put in place to ensure the longevity of clinically important antimicrobials.

Author details

Tracy Schmidt[1,2*], Marleen M. Kock[2,3] and Marthie M. Ehlers[2,3]

*Address all correspondence to: Tracy.Schmidt@kzndard.gov.za

1 Allerton Provincial Veterinary Laboratory, Pietermaritzburg, South Africa

2 Department of Medical Microbiology, Faculty of Health Sciences, University of Pretoria, Pretoria, South Africa

3 Department of Medical Microbiology, National Health Laboratory Services, Tshwane Academic Division (NHLS/TAD), Pretoria, South Africa

References

[1] Mathema B., Mediavilla J., Chen L., Kreiswirth B. Evolution and taxonomy of Staphylococci. In: Crossley D., Jefferson K., Archer G., Fowler V., editors. Staphylococci in Human Disease. 2nd ed. Singapore: Wiley-Blackwell; 2009. pp. 31–64.

[2] Kloos W., Bannerman T. Staphylococcus and Micrococcus. In: Murray P., Baron E., Pfaller M., Tenover F., Yolken R., editors. Manual of Clinical Microbiology. 7th ed. Washington: American Society of Microbiology; 1999. pp. 264–282.

[3] Cunha M., Calsolari M. Toxigenicity in *Staphylococcus aureus* and coagulase-negative Staphylococci: epidemiological and molecular aspects. Microbiology Insights. 2008; 1: 1–12.

[4] Jørgensen H., Mørk T., Caugant D., Kearns A., Rørvik L. Genetic variation among *Staphylococcus aureus* strains from Norwegian bulk milk. Applied and Environmental Microbiology. 2005; 71(12): 8352–8361.

[5] Cunha M. *Staphylococcus aureus* and bovine mastitis: a public health problem. In: Dong J., Liang X., editors. Cross Infections: Types, Causes and Prevention. New York: Nova Science Publishers; 2009. pp. 117–128.

[6] Lindsay J., Holden M. *Staphylococcus aureus*: superbug, super genome? Trends in Microbiology. 2004; 18(8): 378–385.

[7] Sutra L., Poutrel B. Virulence factors involved in the pathogenesis of bovine intramammary infections. Journal of Medical Microbiology. 1994; 40: 79–89.

[8] Barkema H., Schukken Y., Zadoks. The role of cow, pathogen, and treatment regimen in the therapeutic success of bovine *Staphylococcus aureus* mastitis. Journal of Dairy Science. 2006; 89: 1877–1895.

[9] Tenhagen B-A., Köster G., Wallman J., Heuwieser W. Prevalence of mastitis pathogens and their resistance against antimicrobial agents in dairy cows in Brandenburg, Germany. Journal of Dairy Science. 2006; 89: 2542–2551.

[10] Fluit A. Livestock-associated *Staphylococcus aureus*. Clinical Microbiology and Infection. 2012; 18: 735–744.

[11] Vuong C., Otto M. *Staphylococcus epidermidis* infections. Microbes and Infection. 2002; 4: 481–489.

[12] Becker K., Heilmann C., Peters G. Coagulase-negative staphylococci. Clinical Microbiology Reviews. 2014; 27(4): 870–926.

[13] Ibrahem S., Salmenlinna S., Virolainen A., Kerttula A-M., Lyttikäinen O., Jägerroos H., et al. Carriage of methicillin-resistant staphylococci and their SCC*mec* types in a long-term-care facility. Journal of Clinical Microbiology. 2009; 47: 32–37.

[14] Vanderhaeghen W., Hermans K., Haesebrouck F., Butaye P. Methicillin-resistant *Staphylococcus aureus* (MRSA) in food production animals. Epidemiology and Infection. 2010; 138(5): 606–625.

[15] Gandra S., Barter D.M., Laxminarayan R. Economic burden of antibiotic resistance: how much do we really know? Clinical Microbiology and Infection. 2014; 20(10): 973–980.

[16] Cosgrove S.E. The relationship between antimicrobial resistance and patient outcomes: mortality, length of hospital stay, and health care costs. Clinical Infectious Diseases. 2006; 42(Supp2): S82–S89.

[17] Howard B.J., Kloos W.E. Staphylococci. In: Howard B.J., Keiser J.F., Smith T.F., Weissfeld A.S., Tilton R.C., editors. Clinical and Pathogenic Microbiology. 2nd ed. St. Louis: Mosby; 1994. pp. 243–256.

[18] Kloos W., Schleifer K. Isolation and characterization of staphylococci from human skin II. Descriptions of four new species: *Staphylococcus warneri, Staphylococcus capitis, Staphylococcus hominis*, and *Staphylococcus simulans*. International Journal of Systematic Bacteriology. 1975; 25: 62–79.

[19] Kloos W., Schleifer K. Simplified scheme for routine identification of human *Staphylococcus* species. Journal of Clinical Microbiology. 1975; 1(1): 82–88.

[20] Simojoki H. Bovine mastitis caused by coagulase-negative staphylococci [dissertation]. Helsinki: Helsinki University Printing House; 2011.

[21] Euzeby. List of prokaryotic names with standing in nomenclature [Internet]. March 28, 1997 [Updated: February 12, 2015]. Available from: http://www.bacterio.net/staphylococcus.html [Accessed: 2015-03-03]

[22] Capurro A., Aspán A., Unnerstad H., Persson Waller K., Artursson K. Identification of potential sources of *Staphylococcus aureus* in herds with mastitis problems. Journal of Dairy Science. 2009; 93: 180–191.

[23] Quinn P., Carter M., Markey B., Carter G. Clinical Veterinary Microbiology. Madrid: Mosby; 1999.

[24] Quinn P., Markey B., Leonard F., Fitzpatrick E., Fanning S., Hartigan P. Veterinary Microbiology and Microbial Disease. West Sussex: Wiley-Blackwell; 2011.

[25] Sasaki T., Kikuchi K., Tanaka Y., Takahashi N., Kamata S., Hiramatsu K.. Methicillin-resistant *Staphylococcus pseudintermedius* in a veterinary teaching hospital. Journal of Clinical Microbiology. 2007; 45: 118–1125.

[26] Sasaki T., Tsubakishita S., Tanaka Y., Sakusabe A., Ohtsuka M., Hirotaki S., et al. Multiplex-PCR method for species identification of coagulase-positive staphylococci. Journal of Clinical Microbiology. 2010; 48(3): 765–769.

[27] Longauerova A. Coagulase negative staphylococci and their participation in pathogenesis of human infections. Bratislava Medical Journal. 2006; 107(11–12): 448–452.

[28] Lamers R.P., Muthukrishnan G., Castoe T.A., Tafur S., Cole A.M., Parkinson C.L. Phylogenetic relationships among *Staphylococcus* species and refinement of cluster groups based on multilocus data. BMC Evolutionary Biology. 2012; 12;171.

[29] Somerville G., Proctor R. The biology of staphylococci. In: Crossley K., Jefferson K., Archer G., Fowler V., editors. Staphylococci in Human Disease. 2nd ed. Singapore: Wiley-Blackwell; 2009. pp. 3–18.

[30] Wertheim H.F., Melles D.C., Vos M.C., van Belkum A., Verburgh H.A., Nouwen J.L. The role of nasal carriage in *Staphylococcus aureus* infections. Lancet Infectious Diseases. 2005; 5: 751–762.

[31] Graveland H., Duim B., van Duijkeren E., Heederik D., Wagenaar J. Livestock-associated methicillin-resistant *Staphylococcus aureus* in animals and humans. International Journal of Medical Microbiology. 2011; 301: 630–634.

[32] Kluytmans J., Struelans, M. Methicillin resistant *Staphylococcus aureus* in the hospital. British Medical Journal. 2009; 338: b364.

[33] Chambers H., DeLeo F. Waves of Resistance: *Staphylococcus aureus* in the antibiotic era. Nature Reviews Microbiology. 2009; 7(9): 629–641.

[34] Annemüller C., Lämmler C., Zschöck M. Genotyping of *Staphylococcus aureus* isolated from mastitis. Veterinary Microbiology. 1999; 69: 217–224.

[35] Fitzgerald J., Hartigan P., Meaney W., Smyth C. Molecular population and virulence factor analysis of *Staphylococcus aureus* from bovine intramammary infection. Journal of Applied Microbiology. 2000; 88: 1028–1037.

[36] Haveri M. *Staphylococcus aureus* in bovine intramammary infection: molecular, clinical and epidemiological characteristics [dissertation]. Helsinki: University of Helsinki ; 2008.

[37] Foster T.J., Höök M. Surface protein adhesins of *Staphylococcus aureus*. Trends in Microbiology. 1998; 6: 484–488.

[38] Mazmanian S., Skaar E., Gaspar A., Huymayun M., Gornicki P., Jelenska J., et al. Passage of heme-iron across the envelope of *Staphylococcus aureus*. Science. 2003; 299: 906–909.

[39] Schoenfelder S., Lange C., Eckart M., Henning S., Kozytska S., Ziebuhr W. Success through diversity - How *Staphylococcus epidermidis* establishes as a nosocomial pathogen. International Journal of Medical Microbiology. 2010; 300: 380–386.

[40] Goering R.V., Dockrell H.M., Zuckermann M., Wakelin D., Roitt I.M., Mims C., Chiodini P.L., editors. Mims' Medical Microbiology. 4th ed. Philadelphia: Mosby; 2008.

[41] Strasheim W., Kock M., Dreyer A., Ehlers M. Molecular markers of resistance in coagulase-negative staphylococci implicated in catheter-related bloodstream infections. In: Méndez-Vilas A., editor. Microbial Pathogens and Strategies for Combating Them: Science, Technology and Education. Spain: Formatex Research; 2013. pp. 1822–1832.

[42] Mateo M., Maestre J.R., Aguilar L., Cafini F., Puente P., Sánchez P., et al. Genotypic versus phenotypic characterisation, with respect to susceptibility and identification, of 17 clinical isolates of *Staphylococcus lugdunensis*. Journal of Antimicrobial Chemotherapy. 2005; 56: 287–291.

[43] Frank K.L., del Pozo J.L., Patel R. From clinical microbiology to infection pathogenesis: how daring to be different works for *Staphylococcus lugdunensis*. Clinical Microbiology Reviews. 2008; 21(1): 111–133.

[44] Taponen S., Pyörälä S. Coagulase-negative staphylococci as cause of bovine mastitis - not so different from *Staphylococcus aureus*. Veterinary Microbiology. 2009; 134: 29–36.

[45] Otto M. Coagulase-negative staphylococci as reservoirs of genes facilitating MRSA infection. Bioessays. 2012; 35: 4–11.

[46] Vitali L.A., Petrelli D., Lamikanra A., Prenna M., Akinkunmi E.O. Diversity of antibiotic resistance genes and staphylococcal cassette chromosome *mec* elements in faecal isolates of coagulase-negative staphylococci from Nigeria. BMC Microbiology. 2014; 14: 106.

[47] Al Zahrani I.A. A novel multiplex PCR-based tool of typing strains of *Staphylococcus aureus* [thesis]. Newcastle: University of Newcastle; 2011. 228 p. Available from: https://theses.ncl.ac.uk/dspace/bitstream/10443/1171/1/Al-Zahrani

[48] Shittu A., Lin J. Insights on virulence and antibiotic resistance: a review of the accessory genome of *Staphylococcus aureus*. Wounds. 2007; 19(9): 237–244.

[49] Lindsay J., Holden M. Understanding the rise of the superbug: investigation of the evolution and genomic variation of *Staphylococcus aureus*. Functional and Integrated Genomics. 2006; 6(3): 186–201.

[50] Lindsay J.A. Genomic variation and evolution of *Staphylococcus aureus*. International Journal of Medical Microbiology. 2010; 300: 98–103.

[51] Jensen S.O., Lyon B.R. Genetics of antimicrobial resistance in *Staphylococcus aureus*. Future Microbiology. 2009; 4(5): 565–582.

[52] Devriese L.A., Oeding P. Characteristics of *Staphylococcus aureus* strains isolated from different animal species. Research in Veterinary Science. 1976; 21(3): 284–291.

[53] Devriese, L. A. A simplified system for biotyping *Staphylococcus aureus* strains isolated from different animals species. Journal of Applied Bacteriology. 1984; 56: 215–220.

[54] Fitzgerald J.R. Livestock-associated *Staphylococcus aureus*: origin, evolution and public health threat. Trends in Microbiology. 2012; 20(4): 192–198.

[55] Hennekinne J., Kerouanton A., Brisabois A., de Buyser M.L. Discrimination of *Staphylococcus aureus* biotypes by pulsed-field gel electrophoresis of DNA macro-restriction fragments. Journal of Applied Microbiology. 2003; 94: 321–329.

[56] Guinane C.M., Penades J.R., Fitzgerald J. The role of horizontal gene transfer in *Staphylococcus aureus* host adaptation. Virulence. 2011; 2(3): 241–243.

[57] Alves P., McCulloch J., Even S., Maréchal C., Thierry A., Grosset N., et al. Molecular characterisation of *Staphylococcus aureus* strains isolated from small and large ruminants reveals a host rather than tissue specificity. Veterinary Microbiology. 2009; 137: 190–195.

[58] Lowder B., Guinane C., Ben Zakour N.L., Weinert L.A., Conway-Morris A., Cartwright R.A. et al. Recent human-to-poultry host jump, adaptation, and pandemic spread of *Staphylococcus aureus*. Proceedings of the National Academy of Sciences. 2009; 106(46): 19545–19550.

[59] Herron-Olson L., Fitzgerald J., Musser J., Kapur V. Molecular correlates of host specialization in *Staphylococcus aureus*. PLoS One. 2007; 2(10): e1120.

[60] Holmes M., Zadoks R. Methicillin Resistant *S. aureus* in human and bovine mastitis. Journal of Mammary Gland Biology and Neoplasia. 2011; 16: 373–382.

[61] Sakwinska O., Giddey M., Moreillon M., Morisset D., Waldvogel A., Moreillon P. *Staphylococcus aureus* host range and human-bovine host shift. Applied and Environmental Microbiology. 2011; 77: 5908–5915.

[62] Shepheard M., Flemin V., Connor T., Corander J., Feil E.J., Fraser C. Historial zoonoses and other changes in host tropism of *Staphylococcus aureus*, identified by phylogenetic analysis of a population dataset. PLoS One. 2013; 8(5): e62369.

[63] Weinert L., Welch J., Suchard M., Lemey P., Rambaut T., Fitzgerald J. Molecular dating of human-to-bovid host jumps by *Staphylococcus aureus* reveals an association with the spread of domestication. Biology Letters. 2012; 8: 829–832.

[64] Delgado S., García P., Fernández L., Jiménez E., Rodriguez-Baňos M., del Campo R., et al. Characterization of *Staphylococcus aureus* strains involved in human and bovine mastitis. FEMS Immunology and Medical Microbiology. 2011; 62: 225–235.

[65] Lowy F. Staphylococcal infections. In: Fauci A., Braunwald E., Casper D., editors. Harrison's Principles of Internal Medicine. 18th ed. New York: McGraw-Hill; 2013. pp. 386–399.

[66] Argudín M., Mendoza M., Rodicio M.. Food poisoning and *Staphylococcus aureus*. Toxins. 2010; 2: 1751–1773.

[67] LeLoir Y., Baron F., Gautier M. *Staphylococcus* and food poisoning. Genetics and Molecular Research. 2003; 2(1): 63–76.

[68] Cunha M.L.R.S., Peresi, E., Calsolari, R.A.O., Araújo J.P. Detection of enterotoxin genes in coagulase-negative staphylococci isolated from foods. Brazilian Journal of Microbiology. 2006; 37: 64–69.

[69] de Freitas Guimarães F., Nóbrega D.B., Richini-Pereira V.B., Marson P.M., de Figueiredo Pantoia J.C., Langoni H. Enterotoxin genes in coagulase-negative and coagulase-positive staphylococci isolated from bovine milk. Journal of Dairy Science. 2013; 96: 2866–2872.

[70] Vuong C., Otto M. *Staphylococcus epidermidis* infections. Microbes and Infection. 2002; 4: 481–489.

[71] Davis M.F., Cain C.L., Brazil A.M., Rankin S.C. Two coagulase-negative staphylococci emerging as potential zoonotic pathogens: wolves in sheep's clothing? Frontiers in Microbiology. 2013; 4: 123.

[72] Rook K.A., Brown D.C., Rankin S.C., Morris D.O. Case-control study of *Staphylococcus lugdunensis* infection isolates from small companion animals. Veterinary Dermatology. 2012; 23: 476–480.

[73] Kumar D., Cawley J.J., Irizarry-Alvarado J., Alvarez A., Alvarez S. Case of *Staphylococcus schleiferi* subspecies *coagulans* endocarditis and metastatic infection in an immune compromised host. Transplant and Infectious Disease. 2007; 9: 336–338.

[74] Tzamalis A., Chalvatzis N., Anastasopoulos E., Tzetzi D., Dimitrakos S. Acute post-operative *Staphylococcus schleiferi* endophthalmitis following uncomplicated cataract surgery: first report in the literature. European Journal of Ophthalmology. 2013; 23: 427–430.

[75] Coetzer J.A.W., Tustin R.C., editors. Infectious Diseases of Livestock. 2nd ed. Cape Town: Oxford University Press; 2004. 2159 p.

[76] Aarestrup F.M., Schwarz S. Antimicrobial resistance in staphylococci and streptococci of animal origin. In: Aarestrup F.M., editor. Antimicrobial Resistance in Bacteria of Animal Origin. Washington: ASM Press; 2006. pp. 187–212.

[77] Smyth J.A., McNamee P.T. Staphylococci, streptococci and enterococci. In: Jordan F., Pattison M., Alexander D., Faragher T., editors. Poultry Diseases. Amsterdam: Elsevier; 2001. pp. 191–199.

[78] Weese J.S., Van Duijkeren E. Methicillin-resistant *Staphylococcus aureus* and *Staphylococcus pseudintermedius* in veterinary medicine. Veterinary Microbiology. 2010; 140: 418–429.

[79] Van Duijkeren E., Catry B., Greko C., Moreno M.A., Pomba M.C., Pyörälä S., et al. Review of methicillin-resistant *Staphylococcus pseudintermedius*. Journal of Antimicrobial Chemotherapy. 2011; 66: 2705–2714.

[80] Menzies P.L., Ramanoon S.Z. Mastitis of sheep and goat. Veterinary Clinics of North America: Food Animal Practice. 2001; 17: 333–358.

[81] Monecke S., Ehricht R., Slickers P., Wernery R., Johnson B., Jose S. et al. Microarray-based genotyping of *Staphylococcus aureus* isolates from camels. Veterinary Microbiology. 2011; 150(3–4): 309–314.

[82] Hussain A., Shakoor A., Yousaf A., Rehman S.U., Zaman M.A. Clinical and subclinical *Staphylococcus aureus* in dairy buffaloes: disease characteristics and antibiotic susceptibility profiles of isolates. The Journal of Animal and Plant Sciences. 2012; 22(3): 217–220.

[83] Petrovski K.R., Trajcev M., Buneski G. A review of the factors affecting the costs of bovine mastitis. The Journal of the South African Veterinary Association. 2006; 77(2): 52–60.

[84] Halasa T., Juijps K., Østerås O., Hogeveen H. Economic effects of bovine mastitis and mastitis management: A review. Veterinary Quarterly. 2007; 29: 18–31.

[85] Thorberg B.M., Danielsson-Tham M.L., Emanuelson U., Person-Waller K. Bovine subclinical mastitis caused by different types of coagulase-negative staphylococci. Journal of Diary Science. 2009; 92: 4962–4970.

[86] Piessens V., van Coillie E., Verbist B., Supré K., Braem G., van Nuffel A., et al. Distribution of coagulase-negative *Staphylococcus* species from milk and environment of dairy cows differs between herds. Journal of Dairy Science. 2011; 94: 2933–2944.

[87] Howard B.J., Keiser J.F., Smith T.F., Weissfeld A.S., Tilton R.C., editors. Clinical and Pathogenic Microbiology. 2nd ed. St Louis: Mosby; 1994.

[88] Fluit A.C., Visser M.R., Schmitz F-J. Molecular detection of antimicrobial resistance. Clinical Microbiology Reviews. 2001; 14(4): 836–871.

[89] Livermore D.M. Antibiotic resistance in staphylococci. International Journal of Antimicrobial Agents. 2000; 16: S3–S10.

[90] Robinson D.A., Enright M.C. Evolutionary models of the emergence of methicillin-resistant *Staphylococcus aureus*. Antimicrobial Agents and Chemotherapy. 2003; 47: 3926–3924.

[91] Turlej A., Hryniewicz W., Empel J. Staphylococcal cassette chromosome *mec* (SCC*mec*) classification and typing methods: an overview. Polish Journal of Microbiology. 2011; 60(2): 95–103.

[92] Chambers H.F. The changing epidemiology of *Staphylococcus aureus*? Emerging Infectious Diseases. 2001; 7: 178–182.

[93] Lowy F.D. Antimicrobial resistance: the example of *Staphylococcus aureus*. The Journal of Clinical Investigation. 2003; 111(9): 1265–1273.

[94] Jevons M.P. "Celbenin" - resistant Staphylococci. British Medical Journal. 1961; 1: 124–125.

[95] Thomas W.D., Archer G.L. Mobility of gentamicin resistance genes from staphylococci isolates in the United Sates: identification of Tn4031, a gentamicin resistance transposon from *Staphylococcus epidermidis*. Antimicrobial Agents and Chemotherapy. 1989; 33: 1335–1341.

[96] van Hal S.J., Fowler V.G. Is it time to replace vancomycin in the treatment of methicillin resistant *Staphylococcus aureus* infections? Clinical Infectious Diseases. 2013; 56(12): 1779–1788.

[97] Hiramatsu K., Hanaki H., Ini T., Yabuta K., Oguri T., Tenover F.C. Methicillin-resistant *Staphylococcus aureus* clinical strain with reduced vancomycin susceptibility. Journal of Animicrobial Chemotherapy. 1997; 40: 135–146.

[98] Weigel L.M., Donlan R.M., Shin D.H., Jensen B., Clark N.C., McDougal L.K., et al. High-level vancomycin-resistant *Staphylococcus aureus* isolates associated with a polymicrobial biofilm. Antimicrobial Agents and Chemotherapy. 2007; 51(1): 231–238.

[99] John J.F., Harvin A.M. History and evolution of antibiotic resistance in coagulase-negative staphylococci: susceptibility profiles of new anti-staphylococcal agents. Therapeutics and Clinical Risk Management. 2007; 3(6): 1143–1152.

[100] Moellering R.C. MRSA: the first half century. Journal of Antimicrobial Chemotherapy. 2012; 67: 4–11.

[101] Nannini E., Murray B.E., Arias C.A. Resistance or decreased susceptibility to glycopeptides, daptomycin, and linezolid in methicillin-resistant *Staphylococcus aureus*. Current Opinion in Pharmacology. 2012; 10: 1–6.

[102] Cunha M.L.R.S., Ustulin D.R. Antimicrobial resistance in *Staphylococcus* spp. In: Méndez-Vilas, editor. Science against Microbial Pathogens: Communicating Current Research and Technological Advances. Spain: Formatex Research; 2011. pp. 714–721.

[103] Foster T.J. The *Staphylococcus aureus* "superbug". The Journal of Clinical Investigation. 2004; 114: 1693–1696.

[104] Shittu A., Lin J. Newer antistaphylococcal agents: in-vitro studies and emerging trends in *Staphylococcus aureus* resistance. Wounds. 2006; 18(5): 129–146.

[105] Tenover F.C. Mechanisms of antimicrobial resistance in bacteria. The American Journal of Medicine. 2006; 119: S3–S10.

[106] Pantosti A., Sanchini A., Monaco M. Mechanisms of antibiotic resistance in *Staphylococcus aureus*. Future Microbiology. 2007; 2(3): 323–334.

[107] Weese J.S. Methicillin-resistant *Staphylococcus aureus* in animals. ILAR Journal. 2010; 51(3): 233–244.

[108] Tsubakishita S., Kuwahara-Arai K., Sasaki T., Hiramatsu K. Origin and molecular evolution of the determinant of methicillin resistance in staphylococci. Antimicrobial Agents and Chemotherapy. 2010; 54(10): 4352–4359.

[109] Ito T., Katayama Y., Asada K., Mori N., Tsutsumimoto K., Tiensasitom C., et al. Structural composition of three types of staphylococcal cassette chromosome *mec* integrated in the chromosome in methicillin-resistant *Staphylococcus aureus*. Antimicrobial Agents and Chemotherapy. 2001; 45: 1323–1336.

[110] Oliveira D.C., Tomasz A., de Lancastre, H. Secrets of a human pathogen: molecular evolution of pandemic clones of methicillin-resistant *Staphylococcus aureus*. The Lancet Infectious Diseases. 2002; 2: 180–189.

[111] International Working Group on the Classification of Staphylococcal Cassette Chromosome Elements. Available from: http://www.sccmec.org/Pages/SCC_TypesEN.html [Accessed: 2014-11-11]

[112] International Working Group on the Classification of Staphylococcal Cassette Chromosome Elements (IWG-SCC). Classification of staphylococcal cassette chromosome *mec* (SCC*mec*): guidelines for reporting novel SCC*mec* elements. Antimicrobial Agents and Chemotherapy. 2009; 53(12): 4961–4967.

[113] Barbier F., Ruppe E., Hernandez D., Lebeaux D., Francois P., Felix B., et al. Methicillin-resistant coagulase-negative staphylococci in the community: high homology of

SCC*mec* IVa between *Staphylococcus epidermidis* and major clones of methicillin-resistant *Staphylococcus aureus*. The Journal of Infectious Diseases. 2010; 202(2): 270–281.

[114] Hanssen A-M., Sollid J.U.E. Multiple staphylococcal cassette chromosomes and allelic variants of cassette chromosome recombinases in *Staphylococcus aureus* and coagulase-negative staphylococci from Norway. Antimicrobial Agents and Chemotherapy. 2007; 51(5): 1671–1677.

[115] Ibrahem S., Salmenlinna S., Virolainen A., Kerttula A-M., Lyytikäinen O., Jägerroos H., et al. Carriage of methicillin-resistant staphylococci and their SCC*mec* types in a long-term-care facility. Journal of Clinical Microbiology. 2009; 47: 32–37.

[116] Tulinski P., Fluit A.C., Wagenaar J.A., Mevius D., van de Vijver L., Duim B. Methicillin-Resistant coagulase-negative staphylococci on pig farms as a reservoir of heterogenous staphylococcal cassette chromosome *mec* elements. Applied and Environmental Microbiology. 2012; 78(2): 299–304.

[117] García-Álvarez L., Holden M.T.G., Lindsay H., Webb C.R., Brown D.F.J., Curran M.D., et al. Methicillin-resistant *Staphylococcus aureus* with a novel *mec*A homologue in human and bovine populations in the UK and Denmark: a descriptive study. The Lancet Infectious Diseases. 2011; 11(8): 595–603.

[118] Harrison E.M., Paterson G.K., Holden M.T.G., Larsen J., Stegger M., Larsen A.R., et al. Whole genome sequencing identifies zoonotic transmission of MRSA isolates with the novel *mec*A homologue *mec*C. EMBO Molecular Medicine. 2013; 5: 505–515.

[119] Petersen A., Stegger M., Heltberg O., Christensen J., Zeuthen A., Knudsen L.K., et al. Epidemiology of methicillin-resistant *Staphylococcus aureus* carrying the novel *mec*C gene in Denmark corroborates a zoonotic reservoir with transmission to humans. Clinical Microbiology and Infection. 2013; 19: E16–E22.

[120] International Working group on the classification of staphylococcal cassette chromosome *mec* (SCC*mec*). Guidelines for reporting novel *mec*A gene homologues. Antimicrobial Agents and Chemotherapy. 2012; DOI: 10.1128/AAc.01197-12

[121] Stegger M., Anderson P., Kearns A., Pichon B., Holmes M., Edwards G., et al. Rapid detection, differentiation and typing of methicillin-resistant *Staphylococcus aureus* harbouring either *mecA* or the new *mecA* homologue $mecA_{LGA251}$. Clinical Microbiology and Infection. 2011; 18: 395–400.

[122] Kim JY. Understanding the evolution of methicillin-resistant *Staphylococcus aureus*. Clinical Microbiology Newsletter. 2009; 31(3): 17–23.

[123] Lin Y-C., Peterson M.L. New insights into the prevention of staphylococcal infections and toxic shock syndrome. Expert Review of Clinical Pharmacology. 2010; 3(6): 753–767.

[124] Naimi T.S., LeDell K.H., Como-Sabetti K. Comparison of community and health care-associated methicillin-resistant *Staphylococcus aureus* infection. Journal of American Medical Association. 2003; 290: 2976–2984.

[125] Cuny C., Friedrich A., Kozytska S., Layer F., Nübel U., Ohlsen K., et al. Emergence of methicillin-resistant *Staphylococcus aureus* (MRSA) in different animal species. International Journal of Medical Microbiology. 2010; 300: 109–117.

[126] Pantosti A. Methicillin-resistant *Staphylococcus aureus* associated with animals and its relevance to human health. Frontiers in Microbiology. 2012; 3: 127.

[127] Huijsdens X.W., van Dijke B.J., Spalburg E., van Santen-Verheuvel E., Heck M.E., Pluister G.N., et al. Community-acquired MRSA and pig-farming. Annals of Clinical Microbiology and Antimicrobials. 2006; 5: 26–29.

[128] Voss A., Loeffen F., Bakker J., Klaassen C., Wulf M. Methicillin-resistant *Staphylococcus aureus* in pig farming. Emerging Infectious Diseases. 2005; 11: 1965–1966.

[129] Cuny C., Strommenger B., Witte W., Stanek C. Clusters of infections in horses with MRSA ST1, ST254, and ST398 in a veterinary hospital. Microbiology and Drug Resistance. 2008; 214: 307–310.

[130] Nemati M., Hermans K., Lipinska U., Denis O., Deplano A., Struelens M., et al. Antimicrobial resistance of old and recent *Staphylococcus aureus* isolates from poultry: first detection of Livestock-Associated Methicillin-Resistant Strain ST398. Antimicrobial Agents and Chemotherapy. 2008; 52(10): 3817–3819.

[131] Graveland H., Wagenaar J.A., Heesterbeek H., Mevius D., van Duijkeren E., Heederik D. Methicillin resistant *Staphylococcus aureus* ST398 in veal calf farming: human MRSA carriage related with animal antimicrobial usage and farm hygiene. PLoS One. 2010; 5(6): e10990.

[132] McCarthy A.J., van Wamel W., Vandendriessche S., Larsen J., Denis O., Garcia-Graells C., et al. *Staphylococcus aureus* CC398 clade associated with human-to-human transmission. Applied and Environmental Microbiology. 2012; 78(24): 8845–8848.

[133] Smith T.C., Pearson N. The emergence of *Staphylococcus aureus* ST398. Vector-Borne and Zoonotic Diseases. 2011; 11(4): 327–339.

[134] Kadlec K., Schwarz S. Identification of a novel trimethoprim resistance gene, *dfr*K in a methicillin-resistant *Staphylococcus aureus* ST398 strain and its physical linkage to the tetracycline resistance gene tet(L). Antimicrobial Agents and Chemotherapy. 2009; 53: 776–778.

[135] Giguère S., Prescott J.F., Dowling P.M., editors. Antimicrobial Therapy in Veterinary Medicine. 5th ed. Malaysia: Wiley-Blackwell; 2013.

[136] Wendlandt S., Feßler A.T., Monecke S., Ehricht R., Schwarz S., Kadlec K. The diversity of antimicrobial resistance genes among staphylococci of animal origin. International Journal of Medical Microbiology. 2013; 303(6–7): 338–349.

[137] Price L.B., Stegger M., Hasman H., Aziz M., Larsen J., Andersen P.S., et al. *Staphylococcus aureus* CC398: Host adaptation and emergence of methicillin resistance in livestock. mBio. 2012; 3(1): e00305–e00311.

[138] Fitzgerald J.R. Human origin for livestock-associated methicillin-resistant *Staphylococcus aureus*. mBio. 2012; 3(2): e00082-12.

[139] Hiramatsu K. Resistance to glycopeptides. In: Crossley K.B., Jefferson K.K., Archer G.L., Fowler V.G., editors. Staphylococci in Human Disease. 2nd ed. Singapore: Wiley-Blackwell; 2009. pp. 193–201.

[140] McCallum N., Berger-Bächi B., Senn M.M. Regulation of antibiotic resistance in *Staphylococcus aureus*. International Journal of Medical Microbiology. 2010; 300: 118 e000129.

[141] Hiramatsu K., Hanaki H., Ini T., Yabuta K., Oguri T., Tenover F.C. Methicillin-resistant *Staphylococcus aureus* clinical strain with reduced vancomycin susceptibility. Journal of Antimicrobial Chemotherapy. 1997; 40: 135 e000146.

[142] Swe-Swe-Han K., Naidoo N., Mahabeer P., Mlisana K. First detected isolate of glycopeptide-intermediate resistant *Staphylococcus aureus* in a renal unit at a central academic hospital in KwaZulu-Natal. South African Journal of Epidemiology and Infection. 2013; 28(2): 126 e000129.

[143] Thompson K.M., Jefferson K.K. Adaptation to stress: biofilms and small colony variants. In: Crossley K.B., Jefferson K.K., Archer G.L., Fowler V.G., editors. Staphylococci in Human Disease. 2nd ed. Singapore: Wiley-Blackwell; 2009. pp. 109–209.

[144] Garcia L.G., Lemaire S.L., Kahl B.C., Becker K., Proctor R.A., Denis O., et al. Antibiotic activity against small-colony variants of *Staphylococcus aureus*: review of in vitro, animal and clinical data. Journal of Antimicrobial Chemotherapy. 2013; 68: 1455–1464.

[145] Beenken K.E., Dunman P.M., McAleese F., Macapagal D., Murphy E., Projan S.J., et al. Global gene expression in *Staphylococcus aureus* biofilms. Journal of Bacteriology. 2004; 186: 4665–4684.

[146] Madsen J.S., Burmølle M., Hansen L., Sørensen S.J. The interconnection between biofilm formation and horizontal gene transfer. FEMS Immunology and Medical Microbiology. 2012; 65: 183–195.

[147] Atalla H., Gyles C., Mallard B. *Staphylococcus aureus* small colony variants (SCVs) and their role in disease. Animal Health Research Reviews. 2011; 12(1): 33–45.

[148] McEwen S.A., Fedorka-Cray P.J. Antimicrobial use and resistance in animals. Clinical Infectious Diseases. 2002; 34(Supplement 3): S93–S106.

[149] Phillips I., Casewell M., Cox T., De Groot B., Friis C., Jones R., et al. Does the use of antibiotics in food animals pose a risk to human health? A critical review of published data. Journal of Antimicrobial Chemotherapy. 2004; 53(1): 28–52.

[150] Collignon P., Aarestrup F.M., Irwin R., McEwen S. Human deaths and third-generation cephalosporin use in poultry. European Emerging Infectious Diseases. 2013; 19(8): 1339–1340.

[151] Huttner A., Harbarth S., Carlet J., Cosgrove S., Goossens H., Holmes A., et al. Antimicrobial resistance: a global view from the 2013 World healthcare-associated infections forum. Antimicrobial Resistance and Infection. 2013; 2: 31.

[152] Kessler D.A.. New York Times [Internet]. March 27, 2013. Available from: www.nytimes.com/2013/03/28/opinion/antibiotics-and-the-meat-we-weat.html [Accessed: 2015-03-13]

[153] Roe M.T., Pillai S.D. Monitoring and identifying antibiotic resistance mechanisms in bacteria. Poultry Science. 2003; 82: 622–626.

[154] Cantas L., Shah S.Q.A., Cavaco L.M., Manaia C.M., Walsh F., Popowska M., et al. A brief multi-disciplinary review on antimicrobial resistance in medicine and its linkage to the global environmental microbiota. Frontiers in Microbiology. 2013; 4

[155] Henton M.M., Eagar H.A., van Vuuren M. Antibiotic management and resistance in livestock production. South African Medical Journal. 2011; 101(8): 583–586.

[156] Guardabassi L., Courvalin P. Modes of antimicrobial action and mechanisms of bacterial resistance. In: Aarestrup F.M., editor. Antimicrobial Resistance in Bacteria of Animal Origin. Washington: ASM Press; 2006. pp. 1–18.

[157] Mole B. Farming up trouble. Nature. 2013; 499: 398–400.

[158] Mathew A.G., Cissel R., Liamthong S. Antibiotic resistance in bacteria associated with food animals: a United States perspective of livestock production. Foodborne Pathogens and Disease. 2007; 4(2): 115–133.

[159] Shryock T.R., Page S.W. Performance uses of antimicrobial agents and non-antimicrobial alternatives. In: Miguère S., Prescott J.F., Dowling P.M., editors. Antimicrobial Therapy in Veterinary Medicine. 5th ed. Malaysia: Wiley-Blackwell; 2013. pp. 379–394.

[160] Cogliani C., Goossens H., Greko C. Restricting antimicrobial use in food animals: lessons from Europe. Microbe. 2011; 6: 274–279.

[161] Morley P.S., Apley M.D., Besser T.E., Burney D.P., Fedorka-Cray P.J., Papich M.G., et al. Antimicrobial drug use in veterinary medicine. Journal of Veterinary Internal Medicine. 2005; 19: 617–629.

[162] Oliver S.P., Murinda S.E., Jayarao B.M. Impact of antibiotic use in adult dairy cows on antimicrobial resistance of veterinary and human pathogens: a comprehensive review. Foodborne Pathogens and Disease. 2011; 8(3): 337–355.

[163] Hammerum A.M., Heuer O.E., Emborg H-D., Bagger-Skjøt L., Jensen V.F., Rogues A-M., et al. Danish integrated antimicrobial resistance monitoring and research program. Emerging Infectious Diseases. 2007; 13(11): 1632–1639.

[164] Turnridge J. Antibiotic use in animals - prejudices, perceptions and realities. Journal of Antimicrobial Chemotherapy. 2004; 53: 26, 27.

[165] Dibner J.J., Richards J.D. Antibiotic growth promoters in agriculture: history and mode of action. Poultry Science. 2005; 84: 634–643.

[166] Prescott J.F. History of antimicrobial usage in agriculture: an overview. In: Aarestrup F.M., editor. Antimicrobial Resistance in Bacteria of Animal Origin. Washington: ASM Press; 2006. pp. 19–28.

[167] Marshall B.M., Levy S.B. Food animals and antimicrobials: impacts on human health. Clinical Microbiology Reviews. 2011; 24(4): 718–733.

[168] Cefai C., Ashurst S., Owens C. Human carriage of methicillin resistant *Staphylococcus aureus* linked with pet dog. Lancet. 1994; 344: 539–540.

[169] Manian F.A. Asymptomatic nasal carriage of mupirocin-resistant, methicillin-resistant *Staphylococcus aureus* (MRSA) in a pet dog associated with MRSA infection in household contacts. Clinical Infectious Diseases. 2003; 36: e26–e28.

[170] van Duijkeren E., Wolfhagen M.J.H.M., Box A.T., Heck M.E.O.C., Wannet W.J.B., Fluit A.C. Human-to-dog transmission of methicillin-resistant *Staphylococcus aureus*. Emerging Infectious Diseases. 2004; 10: 2235–2237.

[171] Loeffler A., Boag A.K., Sung J., Lindsay J.A., Guardabassi L., Dalsgaard A., et al. Prevalence of methicillin-resistant *Staphylococcus aureus* among staff and pets in a small animal referral hospital in the UK. Journal of Antimicrobial Chemotherapy. 2005; 56: 692–697.

[172] van Duijkeren E., Wolfhagen M.J., Heck M.E., Wannet W.J. Transmission of a panton-valentine leukocidin-positive, methicillin-resistant *Staphylococcus aureus* strain between humans and a dog. Journal of Clinical Microbiology. 2005; 43(12): 6209–6211.

[173] Moodley A., Stegger M., Bagcigil A.F., Baptiste K.E., Loeffler A., Lloyd D.H., et al. *spa* typing of methicillin-resistant *Staphylococcus aureus* isolated from domestic animals an veterinary staff in the UK and Ireland. Journal of Antimicrobial Chemotherapy. 2006; 58: 1118–1123.

[174] Weese J.S., Dick H., Willey B.M., McGeer A., Kreiswirth, Innis B., et al. Suspected transmission of methicillin-resistant *Staphylococcus aureus* between domestic pets and

humans in veterinary clinics and in the household. Veterinary Microbiology. 2006; 115(1–3): 148–155.

[175] Scott G.M., Thomson R., Malone-Lee, J., Ridgway G.L. Cross-infection between animals and man: possible feline transmission of *Staphylococcus aureus* infection in humans? Journal of Hospital Infections. 1988; 12: 29–34.

[176] Hanselman B.A., Kruth S.A., Rousseau J., Weese J.S. Coagulase positive staphylococcal colonization of humans and their household pets. Canadian Veterinary Journal. 2009; 50: 954–958.

[177] Weese J.S. Methicillin-resistant *Staphylococcus aureus* in horses and horse personnel. Veterinary Clinics of North America: Equine Practice. 2004; 20: 601–613.

[178] Weese J.S., Rousseau J., Traub-Dargatz J.L., Willey B.M., McGeer A.J., Low D.E.. Community-associated methicillin-resistant *Staphylococcus aureus* in horses and humans who work with horses. Journal of the American Veterinary Medicine. 2005; 226: 580–583.

[179] Morgan M. Methicillin-resistant *Staphylococcus aureus* and animals: zoonosis or humanosis? Journal of Antimicrobial Chemotherapy. 2008; 62: 1181–1187.

[180] Ferreira J.P., Anderson K.L., Correa M.T., Lyman R., Ruffin F., Reller L.B., et al. Transmission of MRSA between companion animals and infected human patients presenting to outpatient medical care facilities. PLoS One. 2011; 6(11): e26978.

[181] Strommenger B., Kehrenberg C., Kettlitz C., Cuny C., Verspohl J., Witte W., et al. Molecular characterization of methicillin-resistant *Staphylococcus aureus* strains from pet animals and their relationship to human isolates. Journal of Antimicrobial Chemotherapy. 2006; 57: 461–465.

[182] Faires M.C., Tater K.C., Weese J.S. An investigation of methicillin-resistant *Staphylococcus aureus* colonization in people and pets in the same household with an infected person or infected pet. Journal of the American Veterinary Medical Association. 2009; 235(5): 540–543.

[183] Loeffler A., Pfeiffer D.U., Lindsay J.A., Soares-Malhaes, Lloyd D.H. Lack of transmission of methicillin-resistant *Staphylococcus aureus* (MRSA) between apparently healthy dogs in a rescue kennel. Veterinary Microbiology. 2010; 141: 178–181.

[184] van Duijkeren E., Houwers D.J., Schoormans A., Broekhuizen-Stins M.J., Ikawaty R., Fluit A.C., et al. Transmission of methicillin-resistant *Staphylococcus intermedius* between humans and animals. Veterinary Microbiology. 2008; 128: 213–215.

[185] Morris D.O., Boston R.C., O'Shea K. The prevalence of carriage of methicillin-resistant staphylococci by veterinary dermatology practice staff and their respective pets. Veterinary Dermatology. 2010; 21(4): 400–407.

[186] Sanchini A., Pantosti A. MRSA: new troubles from the animal farm. Future Microbiology. 2011; 6(10): 1113–1115.

[187] Khanna T., Friendship R., Dewey C., Weese J.S. Methicillin resistant *Staphylococcus aureus* colonization in pigs and pig farmers. Veterinary Microbiology. 2008; 128(3–4): 298–303.

[188] Lewis H.C., Mølbak K., Reese C., Aarestrup F.M., Selchau M., Sørum M., et al. Pigs as sources of methicillin-resistant *Staphylococcus aureus* CC398 infections in humans, Denmark. Emerging Infectious Diseases. 2008; 14: 1383–1389.

[189] van Belkum A., Melles D.C., Peeters J.K., van Leeuwen W.B., van Duijkeren E., Huijsdens X.W., et al. Methicillin-resistant and -susceptible *Staphylococcus aureus* sequence type 398 in pigs and humans. Emerging Infectious Diseases. 2008; 14(3): 479–483.

[190] Cuny C., Nathaus R., Layer F., Strommenger B., Altmann D., Witte W. Nasal colonization of humans with methicillin-resistant *Staphylococcus aureus* (MRSA) CC398 with and without exposure to pigs. PLoS One. 2009; 4(8): e6800.

[191] Denis O., Suetens C., Hallin M., Catry B., Ramboer I., Dispas M., et al. Methicillin-resistant *Staphylococcus aureus* ST398 in swine farm personnel, Belgium. Emerging Infectious Diseases. 2009; 15(7): 1098–1101.

[192] Hartmeyer G.N., Gahrn-Hansen B., Skov R.L., Kolmos H.J. Pig-associated methicillin-resistant *Staphylococcus aureus*: family transmission and severe pneumonia in a newborn. Scandanavian Journal of Infectious Diseases. 2010; 42(4): 318–320.

[193] Van Cleef B.A., Broens E.M., Voss A., Huijsdens X.W., Züchner L., Van Benthem B.H., et al. High prevalence of nasal MRSA carriage in slaughterhouse workers in contact with live pigs in the Netherlands. Epidemiology and Infection. 2010; 138(5): 756–763.

[194] Smith T.C., Male M.J., Harper A.L., Kroeger J.S., Tinkler G.P., Moritz E.D., et al. Methicillin-resistant *Staphylococcus aureus* (MRSA) strain ST398 is present in midwestern U.S. swine and swine workers. PLoS One. 2009; 4(1): e4258.

[195] Cui S., Li J., Hu C., Jin S., Li F., Guo Y., et al. Isolation and characterization of methicillin-resistant *Staphylococcus aureus* from swine and workers in China. Journal of Antimicrobial Chemotherapy. 2009; 64(4): 680–683.

[196] Wagenaar J.A., Yue H., Pritchard J., Broekhuizen-Stins M., Huijsdens X., Mevius D.J., et al. Unexpected sequence types in livestock associated methicillin-resistant *Staphylococcus aureus* (MRSA): MRSA ST9 and a single locus variant of ST9 in pig farming in China. Veterinary Microbiology. 2009; 139: 405–409.

[197] Battisti A., Franco A., Merialdi G., Hasman H., Lurescia M., Lorenzetti R., et al. Heterogeneity among methicillin-resistant *Staphylococcus aureus* from Italian pig finishing holdings. Veterinary Microbiology. 2010; 142(3–4): 361–366.

[198] Vanderhaeghen W., Cerpentier T., Adriaensen C., Vicca J., Hermans K., Butaye P. Methicillin-resistant *Staphylococcus aureus* (MRSA) ST398 associated with clinical and subclinical mastitis in Belgian cows. Veterinary Microbiology. 2010; 144: 166–171.

[199] Feβler A., Scott C., Kadlec K., Ehricht R., Monecke S., Schwarz S. Characterization of methicillin-resistant *Staphylococcus aureus* ST398 from cases of bovine mastitis. Journal of Antimicrobial Chemotherapy. 2010; 65: 619–625.

[200] Huber H., Koller S., Giezendanner N., Stephan R., Zweifel C. Prevalence and characteristics of meticillin-resistant *Staphylococcus aureus* in humans in contact with farm animals, in livestock, and in food of animal origin, Switzerland, 2009. Eurosurveillance. 2010; 15(16): 19542.

[201] Juhász-Kaszanyitzky, Jánosi S., Somogyi P., Dán A., van der Graaf-van Bloois L., van Duijkeren E., et al. MRSA transmission between cows and humans. Emerging Infectious Diseases. 2007; 13(4): 630–632.

[202] Persoons D., Van Hoorebeke S., Hermans K., Butaye P., de Kruif A., Haesbrouck F., et al. Methicillin-resistant *Staphylococcus aureus* in poultry. Emerging Infectious Diseases. 2009; 15: 452–453.

[203] Schwabe. Veterinary Medicine and Human Health. Baltimore: Williams and Wilkins; 1984.

[204] de Boer E., Zwartkruis-Nahuis J.T., Wit B., Huijsdens X.W., de Neeling A.J., Bosch T., et al. Prevalence of methicillin-resistant *Staphylococcus aureus* in meat. International Journal of Food Microbiology. 2009; 134(1–2): 52–56

[205] Pu S., Han F., Ge B. Isolation and Characterization of methicillin-resistant *Staphylococcus aureus* strains from Louisiana retail meats. Applied and Environmental Microbiology. 2009; 75(1): 265–267.

[206] Weese J.S., Reid-Smith R., Rousseau J., Avery B. Methicillin-resistant *Staphylococcus aureus* (MRSA) contamination of retail pork. Canadian Veterinary Journal. 2010; 51: 749–752.

[207] Kluytmans J.A.J.W. Methicillin-resistant *Staphylococcus aureus* in food products: cause for concern or case for complacency? Clinical Microbiology and Infection. 2010; 16: 11–15.

[208] The Danish Integrated Antimicrobial Resistance Monitoring and Research Programme. DANMAP 2012 - Use of antimicrobial agents and occurrence of antimicrobial resistance in bacteria from food animals, food and humans in Denmark [Internet]. Available from: www.danmap.org [Accessed: 2015-02-12]

[209] Grant J., Saxinger L., Patrick D. Surveillance of antimicrobial resistance and antimicrobial utilization in Canada. Winnipeg: National Collaborating Centre for Infectious Diseases; 2014. 1–31 p.

[210] Watts J.L., Lindeman C.J. Antimicrobial susceptibility testing of bacteria of veterinary origin. In: Aarestrup F.M., editor. Antimicrobial Resistance in Bacteria of Animal Origin. Washington: ASM Press; 2006. pp. 29–36.

[211] Sepandj F., Ceri H., Gibb A.P., Read R.R., Olson M. Biofilm infections in peritoneal dialysis-related peritonitis: comparison of standard MIC and MBEC in evaluation of antibiotic sensitivity of coagulase-negative staphylococci. Peritoneal Dialysis International. 2003; 1: 77–79.

[212] Kavanaugh N.L., Ribbeck K. Selected antimicrobial essential oils eradicate *Pseudomonas* spp. and *Staphylococcus aureus* biofilms. Applied and Environmental Microbiology. 2012; 78(11): 499–411.

[213] Molina-Manso D., del Prado G., Ortiz-Pérez A., Manrubia-Cobo M., Gómez-Barrena E., Cordero-Ampuero J., Esteban J. *In vitro* susceptibility to antibiotics of staphylococci in biofilms isolated from orthopaedic infections. International Journal of Antimicrobial Agents. 2013; 41(6): 521–523.

[214] Goggin R., Jardeleza C., Wormald J.P.-J. Corticosteroids directly reduce *Staphylococcus aureus* biofilm growth: an *in vitro* study. The Laryngoscope. 2014; 124(3): 302–607.

[215] Tremblay Y.D.N., Caron V., Blondeau A., Messier S., Jacques M. Biofilm formation by coagulase-negative staphylococci: impact on the efficacy of antimicrobials and disinfectants commonly used on dairy farms. Veterinary Microbiology. 2014; 172(3–4): 511–518.

[216] Aarts H.J.M., Guerra B., Malorny B. Molecular methods for detection of antibiotic resistance. In: Aarestrup F.M., editor. Antimicrobial Resistance in Bacteria of Animal Origin. Washington: ASM Press; 2006. pp. 37–48.

[217] Bergeron M.G., Ouellette M. Preventing antibiotic resistance through rapid genotypic identification of bacteria and of their antibiotic resistance genes in the clinical microbiology laboratory. Journal of Clinical Microbiology. 1998; 36(8): 2169–2172.

[218] McNicholas S., Shore A.C., Coleman D.C., Humphreys H., Fitzgerald Hughes D. DNA microarray genotyping and virulence and antimicrobial resistance gene profiling of methicillin-resistant *Staphylococccus aureus* bloodstream isolates from renal patients. Journal of Clinical Microbiology. 2011; 49(12): 4349–4351.

[219] Hata E., Katsuda K., Kobayashi H., Uchida I., Tanaka K., Eguchi M. Genetic variation among *Staphylococccus aureus* strains from bovine milk and their relevance to methicillin-resistant isolates from humans. Journal of Clinical Microbiology. 2010; 48(6): 2130–2139.

[220] Arbeit R.D. Laboratory procedures for the epidemiologic analysis of microorganisms. In: Murray P.R., Baron E.J., Pfaller M.A., Tenover F.C., Yolken R.H., editors. Manual of Clinical Microbiology. 7th ed. Washington: ASM Press; 1999. pp. 116–137.

[221] Trindade P.A., McCulloch J.A., Oliveira G.A. Molecular techniques for MRSA typing: current issues and perspectives. The Brazil Journal of Infectious Diseases. 2003; 7: 32–43.

[222] Tenover F.C., Arbeit R.D., Goering R.V., Mickelsen P.A., Murray B.E., Persing D.H., et al. Interpreting chromosomal DNA restriction patterns produced by pulsed field gel electrophoresis: criteria for bacterial strain typing. Journal of Clinical Microbiology. 1995; 33(9): 2233–2239.

[223] Weller T. Methicillin-resistant *Staphylococcus aureus* typing methods: which should be the international standard? Journal of Hospital Infection. 2000; 44: 160–172.

[224] Enright M.C., Day N.P.J., Davies C.E., Peacock S.J., Spratt B.G. Multilocus sequence typing for characterization of methicillin-resistant and methicillin-susceptible clones of *Staphylococcus aureus*. Journal of Clinical Microbiology. 2000; 38(3): 1008–1015.

[225] Wright, J.S. Virulence mechanisms in MRSA pathogenesis. In: Fluit A.C., Schmitz F.-J., editors. MRSA: Current Perspectives. Wymondham: Caister Academic Press.

[226] Koreen L., Ramaswamy S.V., Graviss E.A., Naidich S., Musser M.M., Kreiswirth B.N. *spa* typing method for discriminating among *Staphylococcus aureus* isolates: implication for use of a single marker to detect genetic micro-and macrovariation. Journal of Clinical Microbiology. 2004; 42(2): 792–799.

[227] Malachowa N., Saba A., Gniadkowski M., Krzyszton-Russjan J., Empel J., Miedzobrodzki J., et al. Comparison of multiple-locus variable-number tandem-repeat analysis with pulsed-field gel electrophoresis, *spa* typing, and multilocus sequence typing for clonal characterization *of Staphylococcus aureus* isolates. Journal of Clinical Microbiology. 2005; 43: 3095–3100.

[228] Deurenberg R.H., Stobberingh E.E. The evolution of *Staphylococcus aureus*. Infection, Genetics and Evolution. 2008; 8: 747–763.

[229] Oliveira D.C., de Lencastre H. Multiplex PCR strategy for rapid identification of structural types and variants of the *mec* element in methicillin-resistant *Staphylococcus aureus*. Antimicrobial Agents and Chemotherapy. 2002; 46: 2155–2161.

[230] Zhang K., McClure J.A., Elsayed S., Louie T., Conly J.M. Novel multiplex PCR assay for characterization and concomitant subtyping of staphylococcal cassette chromosome *mec* types I to V in methicillin-resistant *Staphylococcus aureus*. Journal of Clinical Microbiology. 2005; 43: 5026–5033.

[231] Boye K., Bartels M.D., Andersen I.S., Moller J.A., Westh H. A new multiplex PCR for easy screening of methicillin-resistant *Staphylococcus aureus* SCCmec types I-V. Clinical Microbiology and Infection. 2007; 13: 725–727.

[232] Kondo Y., Ito T., Ma X.X., Watanabe S., Kreiswirth B.N., Etienee J., et al. Combination of multiplex PCRs for staphylococcal cassette chromosome *mec* type assignment: rap-

id identification system for *mec, ccr,* and major differences in junkyard regions. Antimicrobial Agents and Chemotherapy. 2007; 51: 264–274.

[233] Milheiriço C., Oliveira, D.C., de Lencastre H. Multiplex PCR strategy for subtyping the staphylococcal cassette chromosome *mec* type IV in methicillin-resistant *Staphylococcus aureus*: 'SCCmec IV multiplex'. Journal of Antimicrobial Chemotherapy. 2007; 60: 42–48.

[234] Milheiriço C., Oliveira D.C., de Lencastre H. Update to the multiplex PCR strategy for assignment of *mec* element types in *Staphylococcus aureus*. Antimicrobial Agents and Chemotherapy. 2007; 51: 3374–3377.